JOURNEY WITH GRANDPA

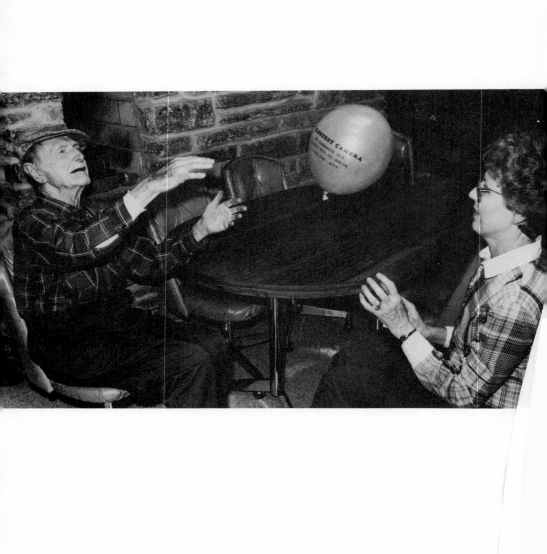

Our Family's Struggle with Alzheimer's Disease

JOURNEY
WITH
GRANDPA

by Rosalie Walsh Honel

The Johns Hopkins University Press   Baltimore and London

© 1988 The Johns Hopkins University Press
All rights reserved
Printed in the United States of America

The Johns Hopkins University Press
701 West 40th Street, Baltimore, Maryland 21211
The Johns Hopkins Press Ltd., London

The paper used in this publication meets the minimum requirements of
American National Standard for Information Sciences—Permanence of Paper
for Printed Library Materials, ANSI Z39.48-1984.

LIBRARY OF CONGRESS CATALOGING-IN-PUBLICATION DATA
Honel, Rosalie Walsh, 1929–
  Journey with Grandpa: our family's struggle with Alzheimer's disease / Rosalie
Walsh Honel.
     p.   cm.
  ISBN 0-8018-3721-9 (alk. paper)
  1. Alzheimer's disease—Patients—Family relationships I. Title.
RC523.H66   1988   88-45415
681.97'683—dc19   CIP

Frontispiece: Press Publications news photo of Frank Honel by Bill Ackerman.
Copyright 1982, Press Publications Inc., Elmhurst, Ill. Used by permission.

For my parents, Leo and Bessie Walsh, in loving memory.

Contents

Foreword

Journey with Grandpa relates an American family's struggle against a devastating horror, the progressive, deteriorating illness we know as Alzheimer's disease. Rather than being a story of tragedy, however, this account is the story of heroism. In a chronological fashion, Rosalie Walsh Honel describes her and her family's struggle and their loving care of her father-in-law through the course of his illness from the early signs of memory loss to death.

What is Alzheimer's disease? Only ten years ago the term was unknown, not only to the American public but to a majority of health professionals. Now the condition is widely recognized as one of the major public health problems facing developed countries in the late twentieth century.

Alzheimer's disease is a progressive disease of the brain. It usually starts in late life and is uncommon before age sixty-five. However, the disease can start in the forties and fifties and, very rarely, even before then. The first symptom is usually memory loss. For several years this is the source of most problems, although changes in personality may also occur. Later, patients begin losing the ability to perform complex activities such as driving, and, over the next several years, they become unable to do everyday activities such as cooking, dressing, or washing. During the last several years of the condition, many patients develop difficulty walking and are unable to control urinary and bowel habits. By this point they are totally physically dependent on others. While this is the most common course, Alzheimer's disease is a variable disorder, and there are as many exceptions as there are typical cases.

Frank Honel, Grandpa of this account, was born in Czechoslovakia and came to the United States when he was twelve. He worked hard and enjoyed dancing and singing. When his memory began to fail in his seventies, he was permitted to remain independent and to live in his own home until he was no longer able to do so safely. In the ensuing years he manifested some of the many common symptoms of Alzheimer's disease: memory loss, wandering, frequent awakenings at night, inability to recognize his family, and, later in his illness, inability to meet even basic daily needs.

The story of Mr. Honel's illness is told with honesty and warmth by his daughter-in-law. What makes her account meaningful is her willingness to share both the frustrations and the joys. She tells of anger, exhaustion, and humiliation but also of the humor, problem-solving, and love that went into his care.

What makes *Journey with Grandpa* important to me is that it is the story of many families. It tells of a daughter-in-law providing the bulk of care; it is the story of what seems to be a rather average Midwestern family and their discovery of meaning in this difficult situation.

Two questions that come to mind are whether the pain and love, frustration and triumph, described here are found in many families, and whether they are limited to America. A comparison with *The Twilight Years*, by the Japanese author Sawako Ariyoshi (Kodansha International, 1984), tells an extraordinarily similar tale of a Japanese daughter-in-law's care of her father-in-law. Clinical experience and a number of research studies confirm that heroic families such as these are commonplace.

PETER V. RABINS, M.D.

Acknowledgments

I want to thank a number of people who helped to make this book possible. Special thanks to a group of writer friends, the Scribblers of Elmhurst, for their honest response and positive criticism: Ruth Christensen, Nan Olson, Hazel S. Dame, Grace Carolyn Dahlberg, Candace Purdom, Maryann Geannopolos, Virginia Novinger, and Toni M. Hormann. Thanks to my instructors and friends at the Christian Writers' Conference, Green Lake, Wisconsin: Lenore Coberly, whose inspired teaching led to my first taste of recognition as a writer, Mary Kimbrough, and Martha May. Thanks to Harper and Row, Publishers, for permission to quote Mother Teresa's prayer from the book *Something Beautiful for God* by Malcolm Muggeridge; to *The New England Journal of Medicine* for permission to reprint "Alzheimer's Disease;" and to my editor, Anders Richter of the Johns Hopkins University Press.

Finally, I want to acknowledge the faith and support of my husband, Milt, and our family, which were manifested not only in their encouragement of the writing of this book but also in the gift of love with which they shared this experience. A special thank-you to my daughters Terese and Cynthia for permission to include their compositions, and to all my family and friends who patiently read the manuscript and/or gave suggestions and encouragement, including: Milton, Cynthia, and Michael Honel, Patricia Walsh-Koci, Elizabeth Walsh-Quinlan, Harry J. Quinlan, Joyce Clarke, and Charles Eichler.

1 · A Man Named Frank

Frank was seventy-five years old, widowed, and had been living alone for several years when he started getting forgetful. He couldn't remember what he had eaten the day before. He kept misplacing his glasses and his money. Sometimes he was hungry and couldn't find anything to eat. He had been shopping and cooking for himself, since his wife had died, but now he was finding it hard to do these things. He was aware that there was food inside the cans in his pantry, but he couldn't remember how to open the cans. He used to know how. Why couldn't he remember?

One day Frank had an appointment to see his foot doctor. His daughter-in-law, Rosalie, said she'd pick him up and take him there in her car, but it was only a few blocks away. He was ready early, so he decided to go by himself. He walked and walked, and everything looked strange to him. He had lived in this neighborhood for more than thirty years, but he didn't know where he was. Suddenly his daughter-in-law drove up and said she had been looking everywhere for him. What had happened? He couldn't remember.

Frank began to worry about his forgetfulness, although he made light of it. "I'll soon be pushing up daisies," he said, but he was afraid that something was wrong with him and that he might have to go to an "old people's home" because of it. A hateful thought.

His son, Milt, and his daughter-in-law wanted him to go to live at their house, but he couldn't do that. Here he had his work to do, his garden and flowers to take care of, his own home. But strange things were happening. Somebody was taking things, stealing his money, his glasses. Once he saw a face at the window that opened onto the enclosed porch. But the outside door to the porch was locked! Frank was puzzled. He told his son and daughter-in-law, but they didn't understand. They thought he was imagining things.

One day Frank had a terrible pain in his stomach, and he started vomiting. He tried to call his son but couldn't find the number, though he knew it was there somewhere. He went outside and saw a young man on the street, washing his car. "Doctor! Get a doctor!" he said. "I'm so sick!"

The next thing Frank knew, he was in an unfamiliar place and there were a lot of strangers around. They wanted him to stay in bed, but he got out anyway, and then they tied him up. He could scarcely move. As he lay there, Frank felt tired. He remembered the factory where he had worked for so many years, and it seemed that his tiredness was caused by his hard work. His feet felt so heavy he couldn't lift them. He thought he was still wearing his high-topped shoes with steel protective plates in the toes. When his doctor came to see him, he imagined that the man was his boss at the "shop." His son explained that this place was a hospital and that the doctors and nurses were taking care of him, but he couldn't understand. Everything was strange and confusing.

From the place they claimed was a hospital, Frank was taken to his son's home. Everything was confusing there, too. The bathroom was always someplace other than where he thought it would be. When he was hungry, people were always telling him he had already eaten. If he had something in his hand, someone would say, "No, don't take that, it's mine." He couldn't understand. He wanted to go back home, but his son and daughter-in-law wouldn't let him. They said he had to live with them now; they claimed it was better for him.

He didn't believe them, and he didn't trust them, either. Where were all his things? Where was his money? They took everything. They had a lot of nerve keeping him here. Didn't they know that he had to go home? Who were they, anyway? Dammit, he had always done what he wanted, gone where he wanted to go! They had no business bossing him. He'd get out somehow. He'd show them. He pounded on the door with his fist, shouting angry words, calling them names. Everyone was against him. No one understood that he had to go home. Now!

Frank was born in 1896 on the outskirts of Czeska-Trebova, a city in Czechoslovakia near the German border. His people were farmers, but there was not enough land to farm, so his father had become a tailor. When Frank was twelve years old, his family emigrated to the United States and settled in Chicago, where two of Frank's uncles had already established themselves. His father found a job as a tailor in a large men's clothing store. He never learned to speak much English, but he was able to support the family on his meager income. There were five children, the youngest born in the United States.

Frank, the oldest, was placed in a second-grade classroom, unable to speak any English. "They made me read out loud," he said, "and I could do it all right. Trouble was, I didn't know what I was reading because I didn't know the words." His twelve-year-old body was too tall for the desks, and he had to sit with one leg in each aisle. He was promoted two grades per year until he was sixteen and graduated from eighth grade. Then he quit school and worked, helping to support the family.

Frank was not much different from the other young people he knew. All from Czech immigrant families, they worked hard for low pay, but they were a fun-loving crowd, and they found time to relax together. Frank bought a secondhand concertina and learned to play it fairly well. He played for the weekly dances that were held at the Sokol Gymnasium (Czechoslovak Society) or in the park. He was a good dancer, too, and he learned to drink beer and smoke and tease the girls. He tried smoking cigarettes and cigars, but finally he switched to a pipe. He could smoke a little bit and then put it in his pocket, and the tobacco was cheap, he said.

When Frank was twenty-one years old, World War I began. He did not have to go into the army because he was not a citizen. At about that time, he began working at a factory that made railroad tracks and rails. Long, thick, heavy sheets of steel had to be lifted and fed into lathes that screeched with deafening, piercing sound. Winter and summer temperatures were extreme. The job paid well, and Frank knew he was lucky to have it, so he stayed in spite of the noise and discomfort.

After several years, he and some of his friends decided to become United States citizens. They enrolled in an evening class and learned about the government and the Constitution of the United States. They had to pass an exam and go before a judge to be accepted. "My foreman at the factory spoke up for me," Frank recounted later. "He told the judge I was a good man and a good worker." He attained his citizenship on November 2, 1924, at the age of twenty-eight. "I am proud to be an American citizen," he often said. "In some countries people cannot vote. I vote in every election."

Meanwhile, Frank continued his social activities with his club, going to the park, where a platform had been built for musicians and dancers, or to the Sokol Gymnasium. Beer was abundant. Everyone had a good time.

"I had a girlfriend, and she was beautiful. She was a good girl, but she turned me down. Instead, she married a rich fellow. She married for money. I never saw her after that.

"I looked around for someone else, and I found Frances. She also was a member of the club. Oh, she was beautiful too, but not so much like the first girl. She was plump and nice, and she had spirit! That's what I like. She liked to dance and have fun. We kept company for a while, and then we got married. I was twenty-nine years old then. Her parents didn't approve of me because I had no money. But I had a good job in a factory, and I was a steady worker."

The young couple bought a little cottage, and after three years their first baby was born. They gave the boy a strong English name: Milton, after the poet. The birth was hard for Frances, the hardest thing she'd ever had to endure. It was a breech birth, delivered at County Hospital. She asked her doctor to make sure there'd be no more babies. In 1931, when the child was three, they bought a two-flat tenement with their savings.

The Depression years were hard for everyone they knew, and many, including Frank, lost their jobs. Fortunately, however, the tenant who lived on the first floor of their two-flat building worked for the transit company, kept his job, and was able to pay the rent. It was enough so that they could get by, with scrimping and saving. During the Depression, people helped one another. They made lifelong friends in those years.

After being unemployed for three years, Frank was hired back by the brakeshoe factory, where he worked at a lathe, cutting steel rails that had to be perfect to the fraction of an inch. Frank was a careful worker, slow and steady. It was dangerous, heavy work, and crucial. No mistakes were tolerated.

He was the same way at home: slow and methodical. Frances was often impatient with him. She wanted him to do things around the house, and he was willing, but he kept his own pace and let her fume at him, shouting her down when he'd had enough of it.

For the boy, this was unpleasant. He remembered all the arguing that went on, and the strictness:

"Drink your milk."

"Don't run, don't shout, don't climb."

"Be quiet!"

When his mother took him to kindergarten, he couldn't speak English, and he cried, so she kept him at home for another year. In the early grades, Milton continued to have difficulty learning English. His parents prodded him to do well. "School is important. Get an education," they said constantly.

Trains and railroads were ever more in demand, making plenty of work at the factory. Frank often worked overtime, and he continued to save his money. Frances was frugal, too, but she'd had a longing to visit her family in Europe. When Milt was ten years old, he and his mother sailed on the *Queen Mary* and traveled to Prague, where they stayed with relatives. They returned to suffer the censure of Frank's family, who accused Frances of being a golddigger. They'd never accepted her anyway. When Frank took the child to visit his grandparents, Frances never went.

With rumors of war in the air again, citizenship became an issue of importance. Frances, too, studied the constitution, learning all she could to pass the exam. She attained her citizenship in November, 1939.

She loved to travel. In summer she and young Milton bused to Wisconsin to visit friends on a farm. The boy was captivated by the openness of the fields and excited by the freedom he was given to explore them. He loved helping with the farm animals and playing with them, and going for walks in the woods with the other children he met there. The atmosphere was free and unrestricted, a contrast to his life at home.

Frank never wanted to go anywhere. He was glad to stay at home, work at his job, and take care of the house. In 1941 he moved his family to Cicero into a small brick bungalow with only slight variations from the others up and down the street, an older home, well constructed, but with deficiencies that Frank corrected over the years.

"Whenever I had a problem I asked my foreman, and he helped me," Frank said. "You see these light switches? When we bought this house there were wires strung all over the kitchen. My wife, she wouldn't stand for that. So my foreman drew a picture for me. 'This is what you do,' he said. 'I'm Union, I can't do it, but I'll show you how to do it yourself.' And I did it. He let me use some tools, and I fixed up the plumbing, too, and built a washroom in the basement."

Milt, an eighth grader at this point, decided to join the Boy Scouts. Here he found an outlet for his interest in the outdoors. With the scout leader's encouragement, he delved into crafts, camp skills, and Indian lore, and went on hiking trips and overnight campouts. There was also Bohemian School on Saturdays. On Sundays he went to the Catholic church service, usually alone. His dad never went to church; his mother seldom went.

During World War II, Frank's foreman approached him with an opportunity. "We need a night watchman, Frank, a security guard. You want the job, I'll put in a good word for you."

"I don't know—why would I want to do that?"

"Well, when the soldiers come back, they'll need jobs, you know, and us older fellas may be out. Me, I'm retiring, so I don't care. But you think about it, Frank. The company could use a good man like you on security."

He took the job and rather enjoyed it. His eyes lit up when

he spoke about it. "I like wearing a policeman's uniform and being responsible for the whole shop. It's not heavy work, but it's important. I walk my rounds in all kinds of weather. I check everything, then I sit and read awhile. Oh, I'm careful not to fall asleep! Nobody watches me; I'm my own boss. I like that. Yeah, sometimes I don't like riding the bus and train late at night, but I have to do it. I'm not afraid; I'm careful. I never let anybody get close to me."

As Milt was growing up, he admired his dad in many ways: his resourcefulness in repairing and maintaining his home, learning electrical, plumbing, and woodworking skills as necessary; his continuing interest in the political process: helping his precinct captain to distribute campaign literature, and occasionally serving as a poll watcher on election day. But the nagging and arguing that went on in their home and the way his mother berated his father made him uncomfortable. He noticed that they didn't sleep together anymore. His dad slept on a cot by himself. That didn't seem right. Milt believed that when he got married it would be different. He couldn't see that his parents loved each other, or him, either. They didn't claim to, and if they did, they didn't show it much. His mother bragged to her friends about the things Milt did—but he felt she didn't really care about him.

They never approved of his girlfriends. There was always something wrong:

"She's not Bohemian."

"Polish are no good."

"Stay away from Jewish girls."

"Why don't you like Dorothy? Her father is a banker."

Milt and I met at college in Naperville, a small but growing community west of Chicago, an area still surrounded at that time by dairy farms and fields of seed-corn. My father was a teacher of agriculture at the high school (under a government-subsidized program to improve farming methods), and he and my mother had recently bought a home across the street from the grounds of North Central College.

I had really wanted to go away to college, but since we lived so close to this one and money was tight, I planned to stay at home for my first two years and then transfer to another school where I could have the total college experience of living in a dormitory.

By the spring of my last semester in Naperville, I had found a small Catholic college in Grand Rapids that sounded just right for me. Milt had transferred the previous January to North Central College from the junior college he had attended in Cicero for two years. That spring we both attended a class for the Catholic minority at a neighboring church, while the other students went to a required Bible chapel on campus. Afterward, on a warm spring day, a group of us—Catholics and Protestants—would sit on the lawn and chat together, testing one another's ideas and our own. It was there that I was attracted to Milt. He was tall and blond, serious and fun-loving by turns, with a warm sincerity and great enthusiasm about him.

After that semester I left for Grand Rapids, but I wrote to Milt, and he replied immediately. The friendship continued and evolved through letters and dates when I was home on holidays and vacations.

His parents were upset. They didn't want Milt to have anything to do with an Irish girl. He lived in a dormitory at school, but during the summer when he lived at home he had to hitchhike to see me. He'd get back home pretty late at night, and sometimes when he arrived he found that his parents had locked him out of the house. Eventually they'd let him in, but once he broke the chain on the door, and they were quite angry with him.

My own parents were taken aback when they got a letter from Frank Honel telling them what a no-good son he had and suggesting, "you fanatic Catholics should keep your daughter away from him." I was not so easily dissuaded.

After graduation Milt was drafted immediately. It was 1951, late in the Korean War years. He had chanced to meet a reserve officer who encouraged him to apply for Officers Candidate School, which he did. This kept him at various army camps in the States, and we continued to write frequent letters. Meanwhile I graduated and took a teaching job in Michigan. With incredible good fortune, a year later Milt received a medical discharge from the army because of a chronic allergy condition that had worsened. We had been thinking about marriage when he got out of the army, so now we both secured teaching jobs close to home, became engaged, and were married the following summer.

The wedding was fairly small, prim, and quiet. My parents invited the wedding party and all the relatives to a luncheon at a country club after the morning ceremony. Later in the afternoon a reception was held in a school gymnasium my sisters and I had decorated for the occasion. Punch and cookies were served. The temperature was at a record high, 104.6 degrees, that day, and there was no air-conditioning, but nevertheless it was a lovely wedding. Milt's parents did not come. The only guests from his side of the family were his youngest aunt, Bessie, her husband, and their two children. We were too happy to care.

Months passed, and though we lived in Cicero within walking distance of their house, Milt's parents refused to see me or to acknowledge our marriage. Milt was chagrined by this behavior, but he said, "Don't worry, they'll come around." His dad began stopping by occasionally, bringing food: eggs, butter, baked goods. We laughed about this, saying that Milt's mother was afraid he would starve without her cooking. When I returned from the hospital after having our first baby, Marian, there were flowers from his parents' garden and some home-cooked meals, but still no visit from his mother. Milt continued to invite them to visit periodically, but there were always excuses. I even telephoned his mother myself, and she spoke cordially to me. When I suggested that she visit, she didn't feel well, couldn't go out— or had somewhere else to go.

Some months after our second baby girl, Patricia, was born, we moved from our apartment to our first home in another suburb. Milt's mother had never seen either grandchild. By this time his dad had accepted me and had even baby-sat on occasion when his mother was on one of her trips. Milt was firm, however, in insisting that he would not take his children to see their grandparents without me. His mother finally gave in. They came for dinner one Sunday in our new home, the animosity ended. However, they would never come when my parents or siblings were invited, so holidays had to be celebrated separately.

For thirteen years Grandpa and Grandma Honel (we called

her "Babi," a Bohemian diminutive) delighted in their grand-children. Two boys and two more girls were added to our family. The children were always eager to visit their grandparents' house. Babi would cook a delicious Bohemian dinner, which would be ready to eat the moment we arrived, at noon on a Sunday. Later Grandpa often took the older children to the corner store with him, or a block farther to the park playground. Other times they played in the basement with Milt's old wagon and toy Zeppelin airship with wheels. When the boys were old enough, Grandpa introduced them to coin and stamp collecting. Meanwhile, Babi and I washed dishes, talked, and tended the baby and toddlers. Grandpa had built chairs at assorted heights so that the children could sit around the table comfortably, and a box of rubber bands or a can full of coins could amuse the little ones at length. In spite of the unfriendly beginning, Babi became a good mother-in-law to me, and I was fond of her. She was kind and generous, willing to baby-sit occasionally, and though she disagreed with some of my methods of child-raising, she refrained from pushing her "old-fashioned" ways on me. She loved each of our children, partic-ularly while they were babies. Her capacious lap was a welcoming place for each in turn. Her Bohemian cooking, meanwhile, was a treat for all of us. The traditional feast was roast capon with bread dumplings and sauerkraut. Babi's special Houska, or coffee cake, was reason enough for a trip to their house, and whenever we visited, she sent plenty of food back with us "so tomorrow you won't have to cook."

Grandpa had many chances to experiment with cooking for himself, because Babi loved to travel. Every spring, for her health, she would take a bus to Hot Springs, Arkansas, with one or two of her "lady-friends," as she called them. In winter she and her friends would go to Florida for two or three weeks. They stayed in inexpensive cottages or with friends, so it didn't cost very much.

Meanwhile Grandpa, still content to stay at home, cooked smoked butt and boiled potatoes for himself and bought rye bread and prasky, a variety of Polish sausage. His tastes were simple and easily satisfied. He was used to shopping because he often accompanied Babi to the store to help her carry things (and complained because she interrupted her shopping to visit with her friends). They had no car, only a shopping cart and the red wagon Grandpa used for heavy loads.

Grandpa had a hearing loss, which he attributed to the shrill clanking noises in the factory where he had worked for over forty years, but aside from that, he was one of the healthiest people I knew. Babi, on the contrary, was overweight, suffered from chronic bronchitis, and complained continually of her frailty and her weak heart. She was hospitalized with pneumonia several times. After Grandpa retired, however, he had a series of hospitalizations himself, for a variety of ailments: detached retina of the right eye, hernia, inflamed prostate, diverticulitis. Each time, he regained his health and strength completely.

The year 1969 was very difficult. It began with one of Grandpa's serious illnesses, simultaneous with the death of my mother, who had suffered a severe stroke five years before. Her passing, though a release from a terrible agony, not only for her but also for my father and my sister, who took care of her, was our family's first experience with death. Visiting Grandpa in the hospital became a reminder of his frailty, too. He recovered fully, however, and in February we celebrated the forty-sixth wedding anniversary of Grandpa and Babi with a dinner party in their honor. In the spring Babi again suffered one of her bronchitis attacks, went to the hospital—and failed to respond to treatment. She died in April, of bronchial pneumonia. The shock came as Milt was in the last stages of his doctoral studies.

We were bewildered and stunned; but the day-to-day bustle of family life with six children ages two to fifteen left little time to mourn. Grandpa was lonely, but he turned his attention to learning to take care of himself. Life went on.

2 • When Surgery Is Necessary

After Babi's death, doing the shopping and cooking for himself helped to ease Grandpa's loneliness. He was really very self-reliant, having often helped Babi to run the wringer washing machine in the basement and to do other household chores such as grocery shopping, dishwashing, and cleaning. Occasionally he would report to me that he had washed his laundry or scrubbed the kitchen floor, along with the other things he did to keep busy. In the evening Grandpa played solitaire or read from his collection of newspapers and *Reader's Digest* magazines that always occupied most of the space on his kitchen table.

His sister Bessie would come to see him sometimes, or he would go to her place. She was a nurse, and she advised him about various over-the-counter medications to take for his occasional health problems. Although she lived within a few miles of him, it was a roundabout trip by bus and city transit, so more often they visited by phone. We had an amplifier installed in his telephone and on his television set so he could hear more easily.

There was a small restaurant on the main street, just a block and a half from his house. We urged him to go there for lunch once in a while. "No," he said. "I wouldn't do that. It's too expensive." We tried to convince him that he could afford to do it, and that it would be good for him, to no avail.

A few of his old friends were still alive, and once or twice a month Grandpa would have a game of chess with one of them, or they'd just talk together about old times.

Sometimes on a Sunday afternoon Milt would drive to Cicero to get him, and he would have supper with us. I would have to serve something easy to chew. A favorite meal was chicken and dumplings. Grandpa would always want to be taken home when he saw it getting dark. He said, "You never know—someone might break in if there's no light."

Many times when we called and asked him to visit, he refused. "It's too far, too much driving back and forth," he protested.

After three or four years, there were changes in Grandpa's behavior, but they were so gradual we were hardly aware of them. Phone calls became more frequent, longer-lasting; complaints more insistent: "I can't find my glasses. Somebody stole them." "My money is gone." "I can't find my bankbook." We would then have to go to his house and conduct a vigorous search of his dresser drawers, pantry and cabinet shelves, basement work-bench, and countless nooks and crannies to find these objects where he had hidden them, probably "for safekeeping."

His next-door neighbor reported that Grandpa was having trouble at the grocery store. He refused to pay for the things in his cart. He thought that the store was charging him more than they should.

He complained to Milt that someone had broken into his house. He said he had seen someone looking in from the porch window. It was an enclosed porch. The outside door was locked. He must have been imagining this.

One by one his friends either died or left the neighborhood. The woman next door said she didn't care to talk with him any-more. "He just keeps repeating the same things, like he's talking to himself," she said. In summer he spent a lot of time doing just that, she reported: sitting in the backyard, talking out loud to himself.

He complained about all the mail he received and worried because he couldn't understand all those "high English" words. I just laughed and said he should throw all that junk mail away. But he wouldn't. He was afraid it was something important, so he saved it for us.

Grandpa had never had a checking account; he paid his utility bills in person. Somehow he continued to do that, and to cash his pension and social security checks. When he didn't know how to do something, such as how to fill out his income tax form, he asked Milt to do it for him. His hiding and losing things was a constant nuisance, but we weren't concerned until he lost one of his savings account passbooks and we never did find it. The bank official very reluctantly made a new one for him. Fortunately, it only happened once.

Then I noticed that he was wearing the same clothes all the time and that they were more and more soiled, so I began doing his laundry and changing his bedding. I would have to get clean clothes out for him and insist that he put them on so I could wash the others. He didn't have an odor, but he obviously wasn't bathing regularly.

It bothered him when I brought my bucket and cleaning gear to clean his bathroom and kitchen. He remonstrated that he "was going to do the cleaning—just didn't get around to it" and insisted on giving me a couple of dollar bills or some loose change "for the children." There was clutter everywhere, but I didn't deal with that.

These changes made Milt and me aware that we were now responsible for Grandpa's well-being. Although he wanted to be independent, he was no longer functioning at full capacity. Therefore it was necessary for us to assume responsibility in those areas where he was lacking.

He gave us little choice. His demands continued to increase.

It was in January of 1977—Grandpa had been living alone for over seven years—when my phone rang and I heard him speaking with great distress in his voice:

"I'm sick! I feel bad! Oh, such a pain! Doctor! Get a doctor!"

"Grandpa, what's the matter? Can you tell me where the pain is?"

"I can't go on toilet. I'm sick. Get a doctor, please! Oh, I feel so bad!"

"Okay, Grandpa, I'll get a doctor right away. You just wait."

I phoned his doctor's office, explaining that it was an emergency, and the doctor returned my call within a few minutes.

"Take him to the emergency room at the hospital immediately," Dr. Johnson (a fictitious name) said. "I'll call ahead and tell them to admit him."

Next I phoned Milt at the office of the elementary school where he worked as principal. It was his first day back after the Christmas holiday. I recounted Grandpa's phone call and Dr. Johnson's instructions. Milt made plans to leave school immediately and stop at home for me so that we could go together to take Grandpa to the hospital. I breathed a sigh of relief, thankful that Milt's job was flexible at times like this.

In less than an hour, we pulled up in front of Grandpa's house, some fifteen miles away. Poor Grandpa! He was pale and obviously uncomfortable, but he meekly got into the car with us and was soon in a hospital wheelchair being taken down the hall and out of our sight. Eventually he was placed in a room, and we were able to comfort him and stay with him awhile.

That evening we received a call from the hospital asking us to confer with the doctor at ten the next morning.

The next day Milt and I were at the hospital before the appointed time. Grandpa was reclining quietly, but his wrists were wrapped with gauze and strapped to the sides of the bed, allowing him about fifteen inches of movement area. There was a restraint around his waist that prevented him from sitting up or sliding off the bed. According to the nurse in charge, Grandpa had tried very hard to get out. So far the belt had held him.

"Hi, Dad, how are you?" Milt stroked Grandpa's hand gently.

"Okay, no use kickin'," he answered with a grin. "I tell 'em to let me out of here, but I can't get out."

"That's okay, Grandpa," I said to him. "Why don't you just stay here until you're all well again? You were in a lot of pain, remember?"

"Okay." His gaze wandered to the young nurse's aide who had walked in and was tending the man in the other bed. "Look, she's all dressed up!" He raised his voice so the young woman could hear him. "You going to see your boyfriend?" He winked at me; she gave him a smile. I could see that Grandpa enjoyed all the attention he was getting.

At ten o'clock Milt and I went to the small office where we were to talk with Dr. Johnson, the general practitioner who had been Grandpa's doctor for about three years. The urologist on the hospital staff, Dr. Novak (also a fictitious name), was there too. We had met him briefly the day before. In a casual, friendly manner, Dr. Novak asked about Grandpa's previous bladder problems, noting that there had been prostate surgery. Milt and I recalled that Grandpa had had such an operation years ago, after his retirement from his job.

Dr. Novak went on to explain that sometimes the body tissues grow back and form a stricture that can obstruct the bladder opening, and that to avoid this, a dilation procedure is usually prescribed on a regular basis.

With some sense of guilt, I told him that I had taken Grandpa to his urologist periodically for a number of years after the surgery, but that for the past few years I had not been taking him. His previous doctor had retired from his practice, and the doctor who replaced him was some distance away. Grandpa couldn't relate to the new doctor, so he didn't care to continue seeing him. Instead of finding someone else, I had simply neglected to take care of it.

Dr. Novak assured us that the condition could be corrected. It had been difficult to insert the catheter, he said, but now that it was in place there was no immediate danger. He was surprised that Grandpa had not complained of having problems before the obstruction had become so advanced.

Milt mentioned that Grandpa had been with us only two days earlier, on New Year's Day. It was his eighty-first birthday, and our custom was to have Grandpa and all of the family for dinner to celebrate together. There had been a Bohemian-type dinner and a birthday cake with candles. He had shown no sign of discomfort.

Dr. Johnson commented that Grandpa was fortunate indeed to have his family looking after him. He went on to say that Grandpa's entrance examination at the hospital had shown evidence of some small heart failures as well as the bladder obstruction. He believed that to subject Grandpa to major surgery at this time might place too great a strain on his heart. He asked if we would be willing to consider a pacemaker for Grandpa.

A pacemaker! This was an utterly new concept to us. Although we had heard of this medical miracle, we knew very little about it. Dr. Johnson explained that the pacemaker helps the heart to maintain its normal beat by supplying an electrical stimulus when the muscle fails to supply it itself. "Let me give you some information to read," he said. He handed Milt a small booklet. "Read through this carefully and talk about it, and let me know what you decide. The insurance that your father has will probably cover the expense, but you can check on that. There is a heart specialist on the staff who will perform the operation if you agree to it."

Somewhat bewildered by this new turn of events, we thanked both the doctors and went back to Grandpa's room to visit with him briefly before going home.

As we drove home we tried to sort out our thoughts and feelings. On the one hand, it seemed that it was important to do what was safest and medically best for Grandpa, and if his doctor recommended this pacemaker, then we should probably give our consent.

On the other hand, we had to admit some reservations about this. Dr. Johnson had a responsible position on the hospital staff, but we didn't know him very well. We had turned to him in an earlier emergency. He was patient and unhurried in his office and bedside manner, friendly and courteous in answering questions. He seemed to have a special interest in heart problems. Grandpa's previous doctor, who had taken care of the family for many years, had retired and subsequently died.

If only we could consult some other doctor before making our decision. How could we obtain an objective second opinion? The difficulty was that, although we had been in this hospital during the many illnesses of both of Milt's parents, our own doctors were several miles away in another hospital, another county. Moreover, the only doctors we had dealt with for our own needs were a pediatrician for the children's illnesses and an obstetrician for maternity care. The school district where Milt was employed had required a medical examination when he was hired, and at that time he had seen an internist, but that had been three years ago. We didn't feel that these men would be willing to help us. They didn't even know Grandpa existed. How could they advise us as to whether or not he needed a pacemaker? Not knowing exactly what course of action was proper and courteous, and having sometimes felt intimidated by curt responses to questions on medical procedures, we were reluctant to pursue a second opinion.

No, a consultation was impossible. We would simply have to decide on the information at hand. But what about Grandpa himself? Would it be best to make him undergo two operations and long hospitalizations instead of one? Were these doctors recommending this procedure purely for Grandpa's benefit, or simply because it was available? How would we feel if Grandpa failed to survive the bladder surgery without this pacemaker?

Several years ago, Grandpa had refused to get a set of lower dentures because he was "too old to get his money's worth" out of it. He preferred to struggle along, chewing slowly, gums gradually toughening with wear. We knew he didn't want any more dealings with doctors and hospitals than were absolutely necessary. Now we told him what the doctors wanted to do and tried to explain the pacemaker to him, but he obviously didn't understand what it was all about. Because Milt was the only child, his signature of consent was all that was needed.

What an immense influence doctors have in our lives! They accept responsibility for our life and death so hastily, so arbitrarily, leaving us either relieved and trusting or anxious and bewildered. What a heavy responsibility that is.

In the end we took the easiest route: we decided to trust the advice of Dr. Johnson and Dr. Novak. The pacemaker was implanted in Grandpa's chest, and a battery was implanted below his waist, just under the skin. After the surgery Grandpa was monitored carefully. He had wires taped to his chest, tubes to his arms, the catheter strapped to his leg, his wrists and ankles tied so that he could scarcely move them. For four long weeks he was confined in the hospital, and he didn't like it at all. Though he got to the point where he teased and joked with the nurses and aides as he had in his younger days, and they were very kind to him, he was far from a model patient. He pulled out the catheter, pulled out the intravenous tubes, and frequently became hostile and belligerent.

Milt and I spent as much time with him as we possibly could. I would visit during the day, and either Milt or both of us would visit in the evening. When he was better, Grandpa was allowed to get out of bed and walk around, but only if someone was with him. When he was in bed he had to be strapped in at all times. On two occasions—once after we had visited him and just gotten home, and again when we had not been able to be there for the evening—we were summoned by the hospital staff because they couldn't get him into bed for the night, even with the help of a policeman. His wrists and legs were bruised and scraped from his constant pulling at the restraints, trying to get free. On the whole it was a very difficult experience for him and for us.

Our life was further complicated at this particular time because Cindy, our youngest child (nine years old) was seriously injured one week after Grandpa was hospitalized. She and Milt had been on a weekend YMCA "Indian Princesses" outing in Wisconsin when Cindy's leg was fractured in a toboggan accident. She was first taken to a hospital in Wisconsin and then driven by ambulance to the hospital in Elmhurst, where her leg was packed in ice until the swelling went down and the leg could be put in a cast. She was there for six days, while Milt and I tried to spend as much time as possible with her, without neglecting Grandpa.

Two weeks after Cindy was back home, Grandpa was released from the hospital and brought to our house, very weak and tired, but happy to be away from all that restriction. We hated to think of having to take him back to the hospital in another month or so, but we had no choice. The bladder obstruction was still there, forced open by the catheter. Once Grandpa had regained his strength, he would have to undergo surgery again. Furthermore, we were told that, although the obstruction could be removed, Grandpa might never regain normal control of his bladder.

Whenever I thought about this, I had a sinking feeling in my stomach. What would that mean? Certainly Grandpa would not be able to take care of himself. Had the time come for him to live with us permanently? How would a man like Grandpa, who was used to being independent and in total control of himself and his surroundings, adapt to living without this basic control? Lord, help us!

As it was, each morning before he went to work Milt had to take care of the catheter, waiting for the first sound of Grandpa's being up if possible, but waking him for the procedure if necessary. The connecting tubes had to be sterilized carefully to avoid infection, and the bag that was strapped to Grandpa's leg had to be emptied. A nurse had demonstrated to Milt how this had to be done, and he followed the instructions exactly. The same procedure had to be done every evening. Somehow there was never any doubt about who would do it. Although Milt was in the habit of leaving much of the care of Grandpa up to me, he assumed full responsibility for this personal type of care: the catheter and weekly bathing.

All of this was beyond Grandpa's comprehension. This "monkey business" with bags and straps and "Don't touch that!" and "Leave that alone!" just proved what Grandpa had suspected all along: Milt was "in cahoots" with all those doctors. They were all against him, including Milt, and it was Milt's fault that all this was happening to him.

Grandpa had always had a love-hate relationship with doctors—even those he liked. He said they were conspiring to get his money. He couldn't see the sense of going to a doctor when he thought there was nothing wrong, for instance, for a checkup or a routine examination. He never refused to go if I set up the appointment—he just let me know what he thought about it. However, when he had a pain, he wanted a doctor in a hurry, and he expected a quick cure.

The question in my mind was, would this twice-daily routine with the catheter have to continue for the rest of Grandpa's life? We could only wait and see—and pray.

Grandpa had survived one hospital ordeal. Now he was to be challenged further by being thrust into our heavily scheduled family, where the pace was much too fast for him and there were many things that were confusing.

Since he was only going to stay with us for a month or so, until he was strong enough to have the bladder surgery, it seemed logical for him to sleep in the spare bedroom on the second floor, the room that our two oldest daughters, now living on their own, had shared. This placed him right in the middle of the morning merry-go-round that would get everyone off to their destinations smoothly—if there was nothing to jam up the procedure.

Grandpa, however, was not used to merry-go-rounds, and he didn't understand the affinity between teenagers and bathrooms. Our mornings began to sound like this:

"Mom! Grandpa's in the bathroom and I have to get ready for school!"

This would be the voice of Terese, aged thirteen, panic stricken. The sound of her loud knocking on the bathroom door would be followed by Grandpa's gruff "What's the matter, for Chrissake?"

"Grandpa, come out! I have to go to school. You can use the bathroom downstairs. Will you please come out? Dad, can you get Grandpa out of here?"

Terese had always had an insistent way about her. She knew exactly how many minutes it took her to shower and dry her hair, and her time was planned accordingly. She made a big sign and taped it to the bathroom door:

> Mart—6:30 to 7:00
> Terese—7:00 to 7:45
> Cindy—7:45 to 8:00
> Grandpa—8:00 to ?

It didn't help, because Grandpa didn't understand. Sometimes it was Terese who was in the shower with Grandpa pounding on the door, shouting, "Lazybones, hurry up in there! I want to wash up!"

Daytime was fairly calm after everyone else left. Grandpa rested a lot, ate often, and otherwise sat reading or looking at pictures. I had to give him a lot of attention, but occasionally I left him alone for a couple of hours at a time and there was no problem.

In late afternoon, when Terese and Cindy came home from school, they talked with Grandpa and began getting to know him. Sometimes, though, even when they didn't want to spend time with him, he interrupted what they were doing, demanding their attention. At dinner, Grandpa had a way of monopolizing conversation, making it hard to carry on the normal sharing of activities. Being hard of hearing, he could not keep up with what was being said. Perhaps it was easier for him to do all the talking.

This became frustrating, especially for Milt, and often caused impatience and anger.

After two months, during which Grandpa's survival instinct and healthy appetite triumphed, we took him back to the hospital for two more weeks of the strict confinement that surgery entailed. It was worth it. The surgery was successful, and Grandpa regained full control of his bladder. Dr. Novak confided to us later that he considered this "miraculous."

After his release from the hospital, Grandpa again stayed with us for a short time, but he kept insisting that he wanted to go home. With some misgivings, we finally agreed that he was well enough, and we took him back to his own house, where he lived alone—with at least one visit per week and supervision by phone—for one more year. We knew we were only postponing the inevitable.

3 • What's Wrong with Grandpa?

During the last year that Grandpa lived alone, Milt and I kept thinking seriously about moving him back with us, but we were frozen in a state of indecision. One reason was Grandpa himself. Whenever we mentioned to him the possibility of moving in with us, he was adamant in his refusal even to consider it. He said he liked being on his own in his own place, even though he was lonely at times. He could do whatever he felt like doing. "I keep busy," he said. He insisted he would have nothing to do at our house. At home he had his wood to cut, his garden to dig and plant, his geraniums and other potted plants to water and care for.

It was true that Grandpa had these things to do, but we could see that he was no longer doing much of anything. His garden had become a pathetic patch of weeds. His house plants, which he had always taken such good care of, were now dry and barren. He wanted to cut wood for us, but he called me again and again asking the same question: "How long shall I cut the pieces for your fireplace?" He couldn't seem to remember the measurement I gave him.

On our part, Milt and I were reluctant to move him to our home because we knew from experience that it would be difficult for us and for our children as well as for Grandpa. We were involved in many activities, with all of us going in different directions at once, and, selfishly, we didn't want to change that. Unlike us, Grandpa was slow and deliberate in everything he did. He couldn't understand why anyone could be in a hurry to do anything. He could talk for hours if someone would sit and listen. Moreover, I knew I would have to be there for him. It would cause a considerable change in my life. Yes, moving him to our home would be the last resort—the very last. I began looking for other alternatives.

Cicero, where Grandpa lived, is a suburb just west of Chicago. It is a traditionally ethnic community, made up of people of Czech and other European ancestry who moved there from the city after the Depression years as their material circumstances improved. The town's population includes a large percentage of middle-aged and older people (18 percent are over the age of sixty, according to *Cicero Life*) whose children have continued to rise economically and have moved to suburbs still further west, leaving the old folks behind.

Taking Grandpa's telephone book in hand to see what community resources there were, I soon discovered a listing for the Cicero Council on Aging. The address given was on the main thoroughfare, not far from Grandpa's home. I telephoned, asked a few questions, and made an appointment to see what the Council on Aging had to offer in the way of day care.

The Council was located in an old bank building, the lobby of which had been converted into a social center. It was filled with quiet activity when I arrived: it held perhaps thirty or more people—groups of neatly dressed, stocky, gray-haired women and a smaller number of solemn-faced men; some sitting in twos or fours playing cards, dice, chess, or checkers; some knitting or crocheting; and some just sitting alone as if waiting. I hesitated, taking it all in, and then I noticed a woman seated at what seemed to be a welcoming table, waiting to offer assistance. She greeted me graciously and proceeded to describe all the activities available at the Council: games, trips, speakers, and daily luncheon at the Social Center here in the front of the building; the Adult Day Care Center in the back, directed by Jane Harris (a fictitious name); and also a meal-delivery plan for people who were homebound. I said I was particularly interested in the Adult Day Care Center, so she directed me to the hallway leading to the back of the building. I found myself at the open door of a small, rather cluttered office where a forty-ish woman sat working at her desk.

She introduced herself as Jane Harris and invited me to tell her how she could be of service to me.

I explained that my father-in-law, who lived in this area, was having difficulty functioning at home alone, and asked what resources were available here that could help him. She described the Adult Day Care Center as designed for people who needed help and supervision. It included transportation to and from their homes and a hot meal. They could attend the center from two to five days a week and engage in guided activity to the extent of their ability.

All of this was a revelation to me, and I wished I had known about it sooner. Actually, I later found out that the organization had been in existence for only two years (since federal funding had become available) and had moved into this building just a few months before.

I related to Jane the difficulties I was having with Grandpa and some of his background: that he lived alone and had a hearing loss stemming from his work in a noisy factory; that he was eccentric about his money—if he came for lunch he would have to think it was free. I described his forgetfulness and confusion, his desire for independence but the gradual decline in his ability to maintain it. I shared with her my thoughts—that it would be ideal if Grandpa could stay at home and receive a hot meal every day—except that with his hearing loss he could not be depended upon to answer the door promptly, and besides I was afraid he would not accept meals from a stranger, even if I paid for them without his knowledge. (Perhaps I dismissed this option too hastily.)

The adult day care program, I felt, was a real possibility. Jane explained that Grandpa could be picked up by a van in the morning, do simple group activities, have lunch, and be brought home again in the afternoon. It sounded great. However, I couldn't imagine Grandpa cooperating with the transportation service, at least for now. I would have to take him to the center and home again myself. It was worth a try. The van had arrived and program participants were slowly making their way into the room, so Jane suggested that I stay awhile and observe the program. I was pleased to do so.

The people were gathering in a sitting area where a number of upholstered chairs and sofas were arranged in a big circle in a large room adjoining Jane's office. As they arrived, they were signing in. Jane introduced me to a younger, heavy-set woman: "This is Lillian, one of our aides." Lillian smiled warmly and then moved to where one of the clients was wandering away from the sitting area. She guided her to a chair and sat next to her. I found a place some distance away where I could sit and watch what transpired.

One of the new arrivals was a neatly dressed gentleman, white-haired and balding, who went up to each of the people seated in the circle, shook hands, and said a few words. Then he sat in the circle and began reading his newspaper, which he had carried under his arm. He looked quite normal to me.

A gray-haired gentlemen, tall and slender, ambled across the room, greeting the people he passed by, and sat at the piano which was against the wall near the chairs. He plunked a few random notes and then began playing "Ain't She Sweet." Soon there were people clapping to the music. He went on to play other oldies such as "Tip-Toe Through the Tulips with Me," "Beautiful Dreamer," and "It Had to Be You." Meanwhile there were more hands clapping, heads bobbing, feet tapping, and voices joining in. I heard a lovely obbligato in harmony which I traced to a woman with stark white hair who moved her torso rhythmically as she sang and clapped.

After fifteen minutes or so of this, the piano player (a volunteer from the Social Center, I was told) left. Another aide, Mary, put a record on the phonograph and began leading exercises to music—very gentle movements of hands, wrists, arms, and ankles—while Lillian took first one woman, then others, one at a time, to the bathroom. It was all very low-key, very subtly organized. Later there would be coffee breaks, craft activities, and lunch. One woman sat alone at a long table which I assumed was used for crafts. She was doing some needlework. Apparently she didn't want to join the group and was not compelled to do so.

Jane came and sat with me for a while longer to explain just what I would have to do before Grandpa could be enrolled in the program. He would be required to have a doctor's examination and a chest Xray; in addition, there were forms Milt and I would have to fill out. Jane said that one of the aides was an occupational therapist, the other an experienced social worker's aide. Jane herself had worked in a religious retreat center for twenty-two years before her involvement here. A nurse came in regularly to check blood pressures and document progress. While I was there she worked with one of the clients, a man who had had several strokes and could not speak. He kept dozing, and she tried to wake him and keep him alert—so that he would eat his lunch, Jane explained.

Thanking her, I left and drove home, feeling hopeful that Grandpa would like going to the day care center, and that it would help him. It would be a nuisance for me to make two trips back and forth to Cicero each time, but at least I knew that Grandpa would be well taken care of for the greater part of the day. Eventually, if he got to know the people, perhaps he could be picked up in the van so that I wouldn't have to drive him.

Several weeks went by before all the preparations could be made. Finally I took the signed papers back to Jane Harris and made arrangements for Grandpa to attend the day care center on Tuesdays and Thursdays, five hours per day, beginning the following week.

Afterward I stopped to see Grandpa and tried to share my enthusiasm as I told him there was "something special" we were going to do on Tuesday morning.

When Tuesday morning came, I arrived at his home shortly before nine-thirty. He was wearing his usual black pants and a tan shirt, clean if a little rumpled. He looked presentable enough. He accompanied me very readily, making no comment about the people gathering around as we entered the facility. We walked slowly back to where the adult day care program took place. Jane Harris greeted us; I hung up Grandpa's coat, and we were introduced to several other people. Everyone went by first names here—I wasn't sure whether they were aides or participants. One of the women was particularly friendly to Grandpa. Her name was Julia. She began chatting with him as if she knew him. Jane took his hand and led the two of them to the sitting area, where Grandpa's new friend continued to talk to him. I saw no reason to stay, so I told Jane that I'd be back at three o'clock and left, feeling very relieved.

Later, when I came for him, Grandpa was in good spirits, cheerful though uncommunicative about the day's events. Jane said that he had participated well and had been likeable and cooperative. I took Grandpa to his home and stayed awhile, making sure he had enough food on hand and listening to his familiar recital of the things he did to keep himself busy. Nothing new. I told him we were going to do "something special" again on Thursday. I was afraid to tell him where we were going because he might take a notion to go by himself and get lost, which had happened on other occasions.

On Thursday we followed the same procedure. I picked Grandpa up at nine-thirty, took him to the day care center, made sure he was settled there, and drove home, returning before three o'clock in the afternoon to fetch him. All went well.

That Friday evening the Adult Day Care Center was having its Christmas party, and our whole family was invited. None of our children wanted to go, but Milt and I picked up Grandpa, and we joined in the Christmas-carol sing-along, listened to various speakers who talked about the program, and met the other participants, eleven in all, and their families. There were craft items on display and handmade ornaments on the Christmas tree, some of which Grandpa had made. Grandpa and the other clients received gifts from Santa. It reminded me of the many Parent-Teacher Association open house activities we had attended with our children. We were pleased that Grandpa could share in this program. He seemed happy about it also.

The next Tuesday I again took him to the day care center as scheduled. Jane Harris welcomed him and helped him take off his coat. It seemed to me that Grandpa was becoming familiar with this place and these people. They greeted him, calling him by name, and he responded with friendly handshakes.

"Goodbye, Grandpa. I'll see you in a little while," I assured him, as Jane ushered him over to where the group was gathering. I left, got my car, and made the twenty-minute drive back home. I had no more than taken off my coat when the phone rang.

"Mrs. Honel? This is Jane Harris at the Adult Day Care Center. I'm afraid you'll have to come and get Frank."

"Oh, my!—What happened?" I closed my eyes and took a deep breath, letting out a long sigh.

"Well, he was fine at first. Lillian was talking with him, but he seemed restless. Then he said he wanted to go home, and she explained that he couldn't go home until after lunch. Well, he wouldn't listen at all and became more and more upset. He kept saying, 'They brought me here so they could get in my house and steal my furniture!' I spoke to him and tried to reason with him, but he was determined to leave. I couldn't let him go alone, so I sent Lillian and Mary [the two aides] with him to make sure he got there."

"I'm sure I'll find them. Don't worry."

"Thank you. I'm awfully sorry about this."

I hung up feeling confused and frustrated. What had happened to upset Grandpa? Why did he think someone would steal his furniture while he was away? Was it just his old hang-up about not wanting to go away on vacation or to stay at our house overnight? His excuse had always been that he had to take care of his house. I recalled the many times he thought someone had taken his money when he had hidden it somewhere himself.

But Grandpa had seemed to like the day care center. I wondered if someone had done or said something unkind to him. It didn't seem to be that. Perhaps he just got tired of cooperating, being acquiescent.

Regardless of the reason, this was a baffling situation, and there were more questions than answers. I mulled it all over as I drove back to Cicero. Somewhat short of breath and with a queasy feeling in my stomach, I arrived at his house. There was no sign of anyone there. I went back to the Adult Day Care Center. Neither he nor the staff persons had returned.

Instead of retracing my route, I drove along the side streets, and eventually I saw Grandpa with a postman, only a short distance from his home.

Grandpa would not have anything to do with me. He was visibly upset and shouted that I was no good and I should "beat it!" The postman said that Frank had recognized him, and that the women who were following him had explained the situation. When he assured them that he knew Frank and would see that he got home safely, they returned to the center.

I was so indebted to that kindly postman that I tried to pay him for his time, but he wouldn't take any money. He said he was just glad that Frank had recognized him by his uniform and felt safe with him.

Meanwhile, Grandpa had gone inside his house and bolted the door. He wouldn't answer my knock. I returned to the Adult Day Care Center, thanked Jane Harris, and apologized for the disruption. We talked about what might have caused Grandpa to become upset. She said some of the other people in the program were that way at times, and that some were on medication that kept them calm. She added that, much as she hated to say this, Frank could not come back unless we could find a medication that would prevent a recurrence of this sort of behavior. It was unfair to the other participants if she and the aides had to give all their attention to him.

Accepting this new turn of events was difficult, since I had counted on day care as a positive response to Grandpa's problem. Now what?

Grandpa was due for a routine check-up with Dr. Johnson soon afterward, and I took the opportunity to tell Dr. Johnson all about the day care problem; how Grandpa had seemed to enjoy the stimulation, but had gotten upset and left on the third day. Dr. Johnson listened sympathetically as I described Grandpa's behavior. I elaborated, recalling his excessive concern about money, his hiding things and not being able to find them, his getting lost trying to go places by himself, and also his confusion and sporadic hostility while in the hospital, which Dr. Johnson remembered well.

"What's wrong with Grandpa?" I asked in desperation. "Whatever it is, it seems to be getting worse."

Dr. Johnson's answer was, I'm sure, the best information that he had at that time. He said Grandpa was "senile" and suffering from "hardening of the arteries"; that, in many older people, this condition caused a lack of oxygen in the brain, which in turn caused forgetfulness and sometimes extremely irritable behavior. He said there was no treatment he was aware of, other than good diet and perhaps aspirin to help the circulation of the blood.*

I was not satisfied. "Isn't there some medication you could prescribe so that Grandpa could continue going to this day care center?" I persisted, "Something that would keep him calm, so he wouldn't be disruptive like that?"

"To be honest," Dr. Johnson said thoughtfully, "I wish I knew of some medication that would help Frank, but there is nothing I would recommend."

Another closed door. After having hope of a program that would actually benefit Grandpa and help us at the same time, here I was back where I had started. Should I try to find another doctor? Jane had said some of her clients were on medication that kept them calm. What could it be? Dr. Johnson hadn't said there was no such medication; he said there was nothing he would recommend. Well, so be it.

I visited the day care center again and told Jane that our doctor could not prescribe anything for Grandpa. I shared with her my feelings of desperation. Because of her work with elderly people, she had a list of names of women, some Bohemian, who would do light housekeeping for the aged and infirm. There was a chance that one of them would be willing to help Grandpa. I went home with mixed feelings of futility and new hope.

It took days—perhaps weeks—before I could motivate myself to begin calling the people whose names Jane Harris had given me. When I did, answers varied from "already employed" to "sick now myself." However, there was one woman who was interested. Mrs. Galbavy lived about three short blocks away from Grandpa. I went to see her a few days later. She was very understanding of the problem, anxious to help, and willing to work just two afternoons per week at a reasonable fee. Could this be the answer to my prayer?

---

*It was not until almost three years later that research studies revealed that Alzheimer's disease in the aged was the cause of many of these symptoms of dementia. This was widely reported to the medical profession and the general public in 1979.

Soon afterward I brought her to Grandpa's house and introduced her as a Bohemian lady-friend of mine who had come to visit with him. After we talked for a while, I told him that she would come again soon, and we left. She agreed to come on Tuesday and Thursday of the following week.

Mrs. Galbavy liked Grandpa and enjoyed visiting him. She brought him some homemade soup, listened to him talk, and she told me they even sang Bohemian songs together. It seemed to be working beautifully.

When I visited Grandpa the following week, I asked him if my lady-friend had come to see him. He couldn't remember. This didn't surprise me, in view of his forgetfulness.

After only two weeks of visits, Mrs. Galbavy telephoned to say that Grandpa was not answering the door; she couldn't get in to see him! She tried several more times, and finally I thanked her for her help and concern and said I was sorry it hadn't worked out. (I was deeply touched when she phoned a couple of months later to ask how he was doing.)

It was also becoming increasingly difficult for Milt and me to contact Grandpa. Being hard of hearing, he did not hear the phone or doorbell unless he happened to be near it when it rang. His house was not very large, but there was a basement where he puttered and cut his wood, and when he was down there he couldn't hear anything. When I visited, I would ring the doorbell at the front and rear and walk around the house, peering in and knocking at the windows to see where he was and get his attention. I had a key, of course, but it was useless because he bolted the doors. (I had explained my method to Mrs. Galbavy, but evidently she was hesitant to be so aggressive.)

In retrospect, Milt and I could have been more persistent in solving this problem. We could have had a new doorbell system installed to include other rooms in the house and basement; we could have changed the locks on Grandpa's house and removed the bolts so that we couldn't be locked out so easily. These ideas occurred to us at the time, but we chose not to pursue them. Milt was reluctant. It sounded like more work than he had time for, and he wasn't interested in hiring such services. I didn't insist. Milt and I continued to visit Grandpa together when we could, while I took care of his basic needs with my daytime trips at least once each week.

When I finally got Grandpa's attention and he let me inside, he was happy to see me and would exclaim that he had been alone for a long time and that "no one ever comes to see me." He seemed to be suffering real pain because of his loneliness. How frustrating!

As I was leaving, he invariably insisted on giving me something: some dishes he never used, or some of Babi's clothing ("still good—you can wear it"). I always thanked him for these things and pretended they were useful to me. In summer he would take me outside to see his garden, and he would pick some flowers for me to take home.

As week followed week, Milt and I worried about Grandpa but didn't know what to do. I knew of no other alternatives. I felt that we had exhausted all avenues that would make it easier for Grandpa to live alone. He complained of being lonely, yet he refused to come and stay with us, even for a short time. Because of our work and commitments it was hard for us to spend very much time with him, and the children never wanted to go with us to his house. He was simply not part of their lives.

Each time I went alone to tend to his needs, I feared that I would not get inside, or that I'd see him from the window, lying on the floor, hurt or even dead. Should we—could we—force him to move? Such a thing was almost unthinkable. Grandpa was very strong-minded, and I couldn't imagine getting him to move if he didn't want to.

I remembered that, at other times when we were faced with a difficult decision, something had happened that made it easier.

Weeks passed.

Then, in April, a phone call came from one of Grandpa's neighbors. He had been washing his car out in front of his house when Grandpa had come staggering out to him, asking for help, weak from vomiting, and very confused. The neighbor had called for an ambulance to take Grandpa to the hospital.

Dr. Johnson's diagnosis was that Grandpa had suffered a gall-bladder attack. When Milt and I saw him, there was a suction tube inserted through his nose and down to his stomach and an

IV tube connected to his arm. Again he was completely immo-
bilized by straps and ties. Weak though he was, he tried continually to sit up. He talked—a steady stream of questions and
pleading to get up or out:

"I can't move, for Chrissake. What is this? What's this for?
Who are they?"

"Take it easy, Grandpa, you're going to be all right. Just relax."

"No! Son of a gun! Help me get up. I can't get up. What is
this?"

"The hospital is helping you, Dad," Milt said. "You have to
stay like this for a while, until your stomach gets better. Just
wait."

Someone walked by the doorway. Suddenly Grandpa called
out loudly, "Hey, you! Come here! Get me out of here!"

It was one of the aides. She came into the room "What's the
matter, Frank?"

"I have to get up. C'mon, get this thing off. I'm going home."

"No, Frank, not now. You be good, you hear? I'll be back in
a little while." She told us that the only way she could get him
to stop talking was to stick a thermometer in his mouth.

"Who is that? They go away. Nobody. Where am I? What is
this?"

"Grandpa, this is the hospital. You were brought here because
you were sick. You have to be patient, and you'll get well." I felt
sorry for him being tied down like that, but nothing could be
done about it.

He spent a week in utter confusion: weak, disoriented, angered by the restraints, unable to understand where he was, or
why he was there, or who the people were that came and went
away again so quickly.

His body gradually returned to normal, but we could see that
his mind was not capable of making appropriate choices. He could
no longer be responsible for taking care of himself. Finally, we
realized that the time had come for Grandpa to move into our
home permanently. This time, we did not ask him whether he
wanted to or not. When he was released from the hospital, we
brought him directly to our home to stay.

4 • The First Year

Once we had made the decision that it was time for Grandpa to live with us on a permanent basis, carrying it out gave Milt and me a feeling of purpose and finality. Together we emptied the furniture out of our "study," the small room on the main floor that had been a combination office, sewing room, and music room. We moved the desk, sewing machine, and piano into the family room, making it more crowded but still liveable. We carried down from upstairs the top bunk bed and dresser which were no longer used and arranged them in the room that would now be Grandpa's bedroom. From there he would have easy access to the lavatory adjacent to the family room. Now Grandpa would have a washroom all to himself in the morning. We congratulated ourselves on having bought a house that was so easily adaptable to having an aged parent move in. Grandpa would have a secluded bedroom, a family room with a table and chairs where he could sit and spend his daytime hours, a semiprivate half-bath, and access to the kitchen and the main floor of the house. We brought his clothes and necessary belongings from his house and tried to make his room a welcoming place for him.

The house was ready; were we?

It had been more than a year since Grandpa's temporary stay with us. During that time, the major change in our family had been that our second daughter, Pat, had been married the previous summer. She and her husband, John, lived in Elgin, less than an hour away. Pat worked as a first-grade teacher. Marian, our eldest, was a social worker. She lived in a small apartment in Aurora, another Chicago suburb. Mike, having just turned twenty-one, was majoring in biology at Northern Illinois University and was home for the summer, looking for a part-time job. Mart was about to graduate from high school and would continue working at the local news agency part-time until September, when he planned to go to the university also. Terese was just completing her freshman year in high school, while Cindy, our youngest, would start junior high in the fall.

In many ways we were a very ordinary middle-class family. Milt and I had enjoyed the twenty-five years of our marriage, having faced the usual family problems: personality clashes, allergies, and a few quick trips to the emergency room. Our family had survived its early childhood and adolescence intact, by no means perfect, but with a sense of accomplishment and progress. As parents, Milt and I could look back at our ineptitude and naiveté and see that we had grown in many ways through raising our children. They had taught us much.

We were about to embark on a new adventure in learning, one that would change us as a family and as individuals. Not knowing what was ahead, we groped our way forward, one step, one day, at a time.

There was a certain novelty about having Grandpa with us. It was May, the days were sunny and warm, school would soon be over, and there was a feeling of freedom and anticipation in the air.

Grandpa was obviously weak and in need of pampering. The nurse at the hospital had given me a list of foods that he should not eat so as to avoid further problems with the gallbladder. In addition, Grandpa had no bottom teeth, and he had false teeth on top, so I had to plan meals that were easy for him to chew and digest. This was new for me. I pored over menus and the nurse's list, feeling frustrated that there were no lists of foods he could eat, only lists of those to avoid.

He slept late in the morning and sometimes took a nap in the afternoon. Gradually he got his strength back and began to look and feel healthy again. On warm afternoons we put some chairs outside and sat together, Grandpa with his pipe, while I wrote letters or did other chores between conversations. When Cindy and Terese came home from school, they visited with him for a while. He loved all the attention.

After only two weeks of having Grandpa at our home, Milt and I left for a Saturday evening out with some very dear friends — and it turned out to be a surprise twenty-fifth wedding anniversary party, which had been planned for us primarily by our two oldest daughters, Marian and Pat, and my three sisters. Our anniversary was not until one month later, June twentieth. We were absolutely amazed at the number of details that had been arranged right under our noses — even to the care of Grandpa. It seemed that the moment we had left to meet our friends, the wheels began to move so that Mike, Mart, Terese, and Cindy could all dress and get to the designated place while our collaborating friends dawdled in delivering us there. The first thing I said after the shock of the *surprise* began to wear off was, "What did you do with Grandpa?"

My sister Betty explained that she had hired a friend of hers to stay with him for the evening, with two small children in tow.

It was very late when we arrived back home to find that Grandpa had refused to go to bed while that stranger and those children were in the house. The children had fallen asleep on the sofa, and Grandpa was watching the lady to make sure she didn't steal from us.

Even after the party, Milt and I still wanted to mark our twenty-fifth anniversary in a special way ourselves. For months we had planned to leave on a Caribbean cruise on June 20th. Now the biggest problem was to find a way to have Grandpa's care secured in advance. I contacted a number of nursing homes but could not find one that would promise in advance to save bed space for him for a two-week stay.

It happened that Grandpa's youngest sister, Bessie, had moved to Florida with her husband and daughter. Knowing that Grandpa's house in Cicero was now vacant, Bessie wrote to ask whether they could stay in his house when they came to Illinois for a visit that summer.

It occurred to me that Bessie and her family might be willing to make a deal to take care of Grandpa for us for a week and a half, and then stay in the house as long as they wished after that.

She agreed, so the arrangements were made. On the appointed day in June, we picked Bessie and family up at the airport and took them to the house in Cicero. The next day we delivered Frank to them, bag and baggage, and went on our way to Miami and Barbados. It looked like a very neat arrangement.

The only hitch was that Grandpa was back home again, and there were interlopers there, trying to tell him what to do. He was "the boss," however, and he let everyone know it, to the extent of almost literally throwing his brother-in-law out of the house. It was a long week and a half for Bessie, Joe, and Elaine.

Milt and I were blissfully unaware of all of this, enjoying one of the nicest vacations we had ever had, and certainly the most luxurious. We returned to find several urgent messages from Bessie, declaring that Frank was unmanageable and that we should come and get him without delay.

This we did, grateful that at least we had enjoyed our cruise without worrying. Milt still had vacation time left, however, and he really wanted to do some camping. It had been our custom every summer since our marriage to pack a tent and other necessities and go away for a week or two of traveling and enjoying the outdoors—free time in summer being one of the "perks" of a job in education, and a pleasure that Milt looked forward to all year long. So later that same summer I found a nursing home in our vicinity, the Pinewood Nursing Home (a fictitious name), that was able to accommodate Grandpa for two weeks while we went camping with Terese and Cindy.

When we got back, we went to the Pinewood Nursing Home to pick up Grandpa, and he greeted us happily. The nursing-home staff had no complaint about his behavior, and we noticed that he was walking with a surer, brisker step than he had had before, evidently from following the attendants around. He seemed to have enjoyed his vacation, too.

Between the excitement of our anniversary celebrations and our family vacation, we began to appreciate the day-to-day challenge of dealing with Grandpa. His sister Bessie was absolutely right: he was unmanageable. It was a little bit like turning a full-grown St. Bernard loose in your house. Where does he go? Anywhere he wants. So Grandpa roamed at will, whenever and wher-ever he wanted. Fortunately, most of the time that was where we expected him to be: in the kitchen, the family room, or his bedroom. He was good-natured as long as his needs for food and companionship were met—and there was no cause for argument. However, he seemed to find many causes for argument. The slightest thing could send Grandpa into a tantrum: having some-thing taken away from him; seeing the lights on in the daytime, or any such departure from the life-style he considered correct; a disagreement over something; the subject of money, which roused unreasonable suspicions in him. He quickly became a fuming volcano of anger. Eyes flashing, he would continue to spout forth loudly shouted insults and abuse long after the in-cident was past.

For me, having Grandpa in our home at this time was like having another baby. It took all my energy, at least at first. Even worse, it came at a time when I had been anticipating more freedom, not less. Cindy was now in junior high, where she was required to stay all day—she no longer came home for lunch. I had been looking forward to having my whole day to myself, as most of my friends did. Ironically, now that Cindy spent the whole day at school, here I was, home with Grandpa. It was a situation I accepted mentally, even though I didn't like it. Now I had to make the best of it.

I also had to give up some of my outside involvements. For several years I had been accustomed to taking noncredit classes for my own enrichment: classes in personal growth, communi-cation and parenting skills, exercise, and crafts. This was an im-portant phase of my adult life—my awakening, so to speak. Most of these classes were held in the morning or the afternoon, but a few were held in the evening. Now I could no longer attend the daytime classes, of course, but I could still participate in the evening classes when Milt or the children would be home with Grandpa.

Another involvement was weekly Bible study at our church, which was only a short distance from home. I thought Grandpa would be able to stay alone for an hour and a half on Tuesday mornings so that I could continue this. After trying it twice, perhaps three times, however, I realized it would not work. Grandpa had gotten into things and messed up or destroyed them during my absence, or else he had become very depressed. I came home to find him hanging his head and asking me, "What's there to live for? I ain't got nothing."

Unwilling to give up too readily, I began searching for sitters. I thought of asking friends, but I hated to do that; besides, they usually were going wherever it was I wanted to go. I inquired about baby-sitters and tried two of those for a while. They lost interest for one reason or another. People who take care of children do not necessarily want to take care of an old person. I finally advertised in the newspaper and received several replies. One gentleman was interested in helping on a voluntary basis— no pay. He came two or three times and then said he was too busy with other things. Others were willing to come for pay, but they needed more hours of work than I was willing to give them. There were two or three women who came a few times but then quit, either because of Grandpa's hostility or for other reasons. Strangers seemed to irritate Grandpa. He didn't trust them, and he didn't want them around. Understandably, the feeling became mutual.

Finally, I came to accept the fact that my place was at home. I gave up all outside activities during the day, except those which allowed me to take Grandpa with me. When I turned my attention to Grandpa, I soon realized that he didn't have enough to do. He complained continually that he wanted to go home: "There's nothing to do here. At home I have work to do. Take me home."

"Grandpa, you live here now. This is your home," I told him.

"No, I want to go to my own home. Can't you take me there? Which way is it? I'll walk."

"It's too far to walk, Grandpa. You have to wait until I can take you in the car."

"I walked lots of times. How far is it?"

"Twelve miles. You never walked from your house to this house. It's too far."

"Oh, yes. You're lying! I walked many times. It's not twelve miles. If it's so far, take me there then."

"I can't take you now. I'll have time to take you in a little while."

"Okay."

Maybe that would help him, I thought. If I took him to Cicero and let him spend an afternoon in his house, maybe he would find out that it wasn't all that different, that there was nothing to do there either. Maybe he'd get it out of his system, as they say.

I packed some food to take with us. It would be like going on a picnic. When everything was ready, I said to him, "Grandpa, I can take you to your old home now. Do you want to go now?"

"No, I guess I'll stay here."

I might have known! I was more than a little peeved with him as I unpacked the "picnic lunch" and went back to finish what I had been working on earlier.

An hour later: "I want to go to my home. Why don't you take me there? I can't stay here. I have to go home."

"Grandpa, I was ready to take you there an hour ago. You didn't want to go. I can't take you now. You said you would stay here."

"You're lying. I didn't say that!"

"Grandpa, this is your home. You live here now."

Generally, things went smoothly when we went along with Grandpa as much as possible. It was when we tried to make him do things he didn't want to do that he got very belligerent. Trying to maintain an atmosphere of constructive activity for Grandpa was a major concern.

Throughout his life, Grandpa's whole self-concept had seemed to be based on work: keeping busy, being useful. Years earlier, he had spoken over and over about the odd jobs he would do after his retirement. He would never be content to sit around. He cited friends who had done that, and they were already dead. During all the years he worked at the factory, he never took a vacation except to stay home and work on the house or his pet projects. Only once can I remember his actually taking a bus to Florida for two weeks—but it was because a friend of his was building a house there and had asked for help.

Keeping busy, as defined by Grandpa in the years I knew him, meant any of various tasks that he chose to do, such as making a sandbox for the grandchildren, working in his garden, or going shopping. There had to be some semblance of accomplishment or helpfulness.

Perhaps there was a strain of that in me, also, because I always kept on the move from one place to another in the house, from bedrooms to kitchen to family room and back again. Now that Grandpa had moved in with us, I could count on his following me wherever I went, trying to keep up with me. He was very slow, but he wanted to be helpful. When I used the vacuum cleaner, he would hold the cord for me or move furniture so I could clean behind or underneath. Actually he was getting in the way; he wasn't much help, and he realized it. He wanted to wash the dishes after dinner. Sometimes he'd go to the sink and start washing while the rest of the family were lingering after dessert. We hated to discourage him, but he didn't do a thorough job. It was a challenge to maneuver him out of the way and to get him to wipe the dishes instead. There were other tasks he could do: I would ask him to sweep the floor, to peel a few potatoes or apples (this he did slowly and carefully with only a paring knife), or to fold the clean towels as I sorted the laundry. But he made occasional comments that let me know he felt this type of work was "women's work," and he would like to do some "men's work." He even asked if I could get him an outside job somewhere.

The one job he had been working on at his home during the years since Babi had died was cutting scrap wood and boxing it for us to burn in our fireplace. He had accumulated great stacks of old wood, painted and unpainted. Whenever a neighbor would remodel his house or tear off a porch, Frank would carry home discarded pieces of wood of assorted shapes and sizes; he stored them in his garage and all through his basement. These became the raw material for a small table, a kitchen cupboard, stools for the grandchildren to sit on, or whatever simple carpentry he might conceive of; and the leftover scrap wood could be burned. The house was now vacant (later our daughter Marian moved in), but the scrap lumber was still cluttering up the place. So we began hauling loads of wood from his house and giving him a few pieces at a time to cut with his handsaw. Routinely, Grandpa would ask if there was something he could do, and I would say, "You can cut up some wood if you want to." Since it was summertime, he would do this outside on our carport. Milt put two sawhorses out there, and Grandpa would bend over the job, pencil on his ear, adjust his clamp to hold the wood steady, mark where to cut, then place his saw and with a slow, steady rhythm cut piece after piece into one- or two-foot lengths and stack them neatly in boxes. He spent much of his time coming into the house with his ruler and his saw, asking me what length he should cut, measuring and remeasuring.

Sometimes the wood was hard or thick; then he complained that the saw wasn't sharp, or he became overtired and grumbled that he wouldn't do this job any more. On hot days he was irritable and easily exasperated, yet seemingly compelled to continue cutting wood. Seeing Mike sitting around reading a book or having a snack would make him angry. "Why don't you do the cutting? You're lazy, that's what!"

Mike would explain patiently that Grandpa didn't need to cut wood if he was tired.

"Huh! That's what you think! Then who will do it? Nobody. You could do it. You're lazy! You're no good!"

Mike would try to distract him with talk about something else. "I'm going to work in the garden today, Grandpa. I'm going to pick vegetables."

"Yeah? I used to have a garden. I grew vegetables too. Lots of them!" and his thoughts would ramble in that direction for a while.

Always he talked out loud to himself. I could tell if something was bothering him. He would work for a half hour or so and then wander about seeking food or something else to do. Later he would go back to his cutting.

As summer turned to fall and the days began getting cold, he worried out loud about what he would do when it was too cold to cut outside. I was concerned about this also. I considered clearing a space in the basement for him to use, but feared that he would not be able to use the stairs safely, especially with his habit of coming in constantly to check with me or take a break.

It was such a dirty job, I hated to think of having to install his sawbench in the foyer. He had done this, at times setting his piece of wood up on the stone planter by the front entrance, to start his cut there before going outside. That bothered me because it made sawdust on the floor, and also because of his messy smoking habits: cleaning out his pipe in the planter and spitting on the floor! I had already taken the large plant out of the planter because he had broken off several pieces of it. But where could he go? The family room was simply too crowded already. We had to find a workplace for Grandpa that both he and I could be comfortable with.

Finally he gave me the answer himself. "When it's cold," he said, "I could cut here or here." He indicated the planter area in the foyer, and his bedroom, which was adjacent to the foyer. I don't know why, but I had not thought of his bedroom as a possible workshop. (I know I wouldn't want anyone smoking and sawing in my bedroom!) Now I realized it was an obvious solution.

I cleared off the small table in his room. Actually it was one he had built long ago. It had two shelves and a small drawer, and the sides were recessed, leaving an overhang where he could fasten his clamp. From then on, this was his sawbench. When he wanted to do his cutting, I would bring a long piece of wood from outside for him, and he would clamp it on his bench. He was content to have his own space, his workshop. I was satisfied that he could mess up the floor and smoke his pipe whenever he wished, in his own room.

Other problems were not so easy to solve. Milt and I both found Grandpa's sleep habits to be a source of annoyance. For us, the workday morning began at seven o'clock, which gave ample time for Milt to dress, have a quick breakfast, and leave for the office, only a five-minute drive away. Cindy and Terese capably took care of their own needs (as did Mike and Mart, when they were at home), while I moved slowly along as facilitator. Grandpa, however, once he regained his strength, was waking up for the day at five o'clock. He claimed to be quiet so as not to waken anyone else, but instead he talked to himself, very audibly, disturbing those of us trying to sleep upstairs. Besides that, he would get into things that belonged to others, or he would want company and loudly call, "Anybody here?" up the stairs to waken us.

The rest of the family didn't seem to be affected by all this, except when Milt or I failed to respond quickly enough and someone would call out from his or her cozy cocoon, "Mom—Dad, Grandpa's awake," a reminder for us to do something about it.

I discovered that I could leave a snack for Grandpa on the table at night, so he would busy himself with eating when he woke up and not bother us for a while longer. An apple would take about a half hour for him to eat, with no lower teeth and an upper false plate.

After he finished eating the apple, he would start talking to himself again, and Milt or I would have to go downstairs several times to fix something else for him to eat or to find other things to capture his attention so that he wouldn't get into trouble. On weekends it was impossible to sleep in.

Another area where I had to adjust to Grandpa's ways was the evening meal. Dinnertime was the one time of day when we all sat down together. I liked it to be a pleasant time, conducive to sharing the day's happenings, thoughts, and feelings, the delight of being family. I enjoyed setting the table nicely, perhaps having a flower arrangement or candle in the center, and making the meal attractive.

Now I found that Grandpa grabbed at things, so that I could place only essentials on the table. I could no longer use serving dishes because Grandpa would take food from them inappropriately. Instead I began leaving food in the pots on the stove and having everyone serve himself or herself. Grandpa was given one plate and one spoon at a time. I cut his food for him. He ate slowly and methodically, scraping every last morsel from his plate but interacting with the family occasionally. One late-summer evening, our married daughter, Pat, was having dinner with us. I had made a blueberry pie for dessert. It was everybody's favorite. Terese (aged 14) finished her piece and disappeared from the table briefly, returning with a super-clean plate. Pat noticed this and teased her about licking her plate. Then, laughing, Pat picked hers up to do the same. Her father scolded her, saying, "That's not good manners."

Grandpa caught on to what was going on, and said, "I can't get it all with the spoon, and it's so good."

He picked up his plate, too, but Milt said, "No!" in a very loud voice.

"Go ahead, Grandpa, lick it!" said Terese, while the children and I were grinning at him, watching what he would do.

Then I said, "I'll hide his eyes, Grandpa, go ahead!" So I reached over and put my hand over Milt's eyes, and Grandpa picked up his plate and licked it. Everybody laughed, including Grandpa and Milt.

Grandpa's alertness to what went on around him at the table varied from time to time, but in general he was just himself and did what he felt like doing. He ignored us, interrupting what was being said (he probably could neither hear nor understand much of it) by voicing his comments or questions—breaking the train of thought, demanding attention and recognition.

When dinner was ready, we would sit around the table and hold hands, as was our custom, while Milt led our grace before meals.

"Thank you, Lord, for this day, for all our blessings."

"What's that for?" would come Grandpa's booming voice, while Terese and Cindy, on either side of him, smiled, shrugged, or otherwise tried to hold his hands and ignore his voice.

"Bless our family, especially my dad, and help us to be patient . . ."

"I don't want that! No!"

"And bless our friends . . ."

"Where's the food? I'm hungry!"

"Let's pray together."

All of us would join in at this point: "Bless us, O Lord, and these, Thy gifts, which we are about to receive from Thy bounty, through Christ, our Lord. Amen."

"Ahhhh . . . Yah," a great long sigh from Grandpa as we finally finished and got around to the business at hand. I would place his plate in front of him as everyone else got up to fill theirs.

About the time we settled down to have a few bites and some conversation, Grandpa would be ready to interrupt again.

"What's new at school today, Milt?" I would ask.

"Oh, I had an interesting talk with . . ."

"What have you got?" Grandpa would ask Terese, thinking that her plate held something that looked different from what he had. He would take a spoonful from his plate and put it on hers—or try to. "It's good! You can have it!"

"No thanks, Grandpa. That's yours. I have some already. I have enough!"

Meanwhile any topic of conversation that might have been started would be hopelessly lost. Similar incidents would occur sporadically throughout the meal.

Just as disconcerting was Grandpa's childish way of opening his mouth when he had a mouthful of chewed food to show us all "what I got!"

From day to day, as we tried to adjust to having Grandpa in our home, we found we could no longer assume that articles of clothing, school materials, and other possessions would stay where we placed them—especially if they were within Grandpa's sight and reach. He was used to having everything in his home to himself, and so were we. Yet this was his new home, and we expected him to know what he could touch and what he could not. None of us was inclined to change our way of doing things, yet when he failed to abide by our rules we thought of him as an intruder.

One day, Cindy was practicing her piano lesson while Grandpa sat outside smoking his pipe. He came into the house, placed his pipe carefully on the stone planter by the front door to cool, and shuffled over to the piano. Seeing Cindy's small lesson notebook on the bench beside her, he picked it up and put it in his pocket.

"That's mine, Grandpa. Can I have it?"

"What? I don't know what you mean."

"You just took my notebook, and I need it to practice my lesson. Can I have it back?"

"I ain't got nothing."

"It's in your pocket. Look and see."

He reached in the left pocket first, which was empty; then the other. "Is this what you want? Here, take it. They take everything."

"Yes, Grandpa. Thank you." She went back to her practicing. He wandered over to the table and rearranged the papers there, picking up a pencil and putting it in his pocket. Then he proceeded to the kitchen, where Terese was talking on the telephone, her legs stretched out and stockinged feet on another chair. The long cord hung like the top of a barbed wire fence that Grandpa had to lift in order to pass under.

"Is that the way you sit?" he asked, annoyed. "You're supposed to put your feet on the floor. For Chrissake!"

Terese ignored him and went on with her phone conversation. He walked across the room to where she had kicked off her sneakers and left them. Picking up one shoe in each hand, he shuffled back around her, under the wire, down the three steps to the hall, and into his bedroom.

"Grandpa, those are my shoes!" She ran after him and made a grab for the shoes, which he was in the act of placing in his dresser drawer.

"No! You can't! That's mine!"

"No, Grandpa, they're mine. Look, they're much too small for you, see?" She held one next to his foot.

"You people are no good. You take everything." He came back into the family room, where I had just set a basket of laundry from the dryer while I filled the washing machine with the next load. He picked up the bright lavender blouse from the top of the pile and proceeded to roll it into a small bundle and stuff it into his pocket.

"Grandpa, you can't have that," I said, realizing that it would probably start an argument.

"It's mine!" he said with a scowl.

"Grandpa, we're glad to have you living here with us, but you have to understand that we have all of our belongings here as well as yours. You can have your things, okay? That was my blouse that you put in your pocket. May I have it, please?"

"No! It's mine! You people are no good. You take everything. Why don't you go home?"

Anger surged over me, and I grabbed for the blouse. His arm clamped down automatically over his pocket, but I tussled with him, pulling at his arm until I succeeded in getting the blouse away from him.

"You steal! I hate you!" he yelled, as I picked up the basket of clothes and fled, my victory now feeling empty as guilt and remorse set in.

"Why didn't I just let him have it? I could always get it back later," I said to myself. I was ashamed for letting Cindy see me lose my temper. "What's wrong? What's happening to me?" I went back to the family room. Cindy was still busy at the keyboard. Grandpa had found his pipe and was going outside for a smoke.

"Well, I sure blew my top that time, didn't I?" I said to Cindy. "It must be terribly confusing for Grandpa. There are so many of us. Now he thinks this is his home and we are the intruders." We chuckled over the irony of it.

Grandpa had no trouble venting his feelings. He did so primarily with vulgar language, which burst forth in a monologue whenever anything irritated him, which was almost constantly. It bothered me that not only did I have to listen to this, but the children did also. I knew that they would probably hear these things elsewhere, and that it most likely would not affect the way they spoke—but it seemed unfair that they should be subjected to such vulgar, profane talk on a regular basis in their own home.

One subject that aroused strong feelings, especially in Grandpa, was money. We had to learn to steer conversations away from any reference to the topic. But often he brought it up himself.

On one such occasion, Grandpa was standing in front of his dresser, rummaging through the drawers, all the while talking to himself in some of his less savory language. I went in to see what the fuss was about.

"They take everything. They steal. I ain't got nothing."

"What are you looking for, Grandpa?"

"They take all my money. I ain't got nothing; the bastar's take it all. See? Look, that's all I got!" He reached in his pants pocket, pulling out pieces of paper, rubber bands, string.

"Grandpa, you don't need your money here. We give you everything you need; you don't have to go to stores anymore."

"Oh yeah? That's what you think! They steal it. They take everything."

"Grandpa, your money is in the bank. It's safe there until you need it."

"I don't believe you. Banks are no good. They steal. I want my money. I need it. Bastar'! Where is it?"

"Grandpa, I don't have your money. I told you. It's in the bank."

"You're lying! Son of a bitch, I'll find it myself." He started for the door.

"No, Grandpa, stay here. Come, I'll get you something to eat."

"No! I'm going." Out the door he went, and I followed him on one of his countless trips down the street.

Conversation with Grandpa was a one-sided exercise in patient listening. I often said that talking to Grandpa was like talking to a tape recorder. If the word "car" was mentioned, for example, and whenever we got into the car to go anywhere, he invariably came out with: "I never had a car. My wife, she wanted me to buy one. I had enough money, but I saw all the traffic. So I told her, 'Okay, I'll buy a car, but you drive it.' She didn't like that; she didn't want to drive, so I never bought a car." His response was so automatic that the monologue was almost the same every time.

On swearing and drinking: "I don't swear. Some people, they swear all the time, then they go to confession and they say it's okay. I never swear, and I don't get drunk. I drink beer; no hard stuff. My friends, they used to drink and swear. I don't do that. I don't swear."

Sometimes I confronted him. "What about when you're mad, Grandpa, then what do you say?"

"Well, maybe once in a while I might swear, if something goes wrong."

"I hear you swearing and using vulgar language a lot of times."

"No! I don't swear. Get out of here!"

Almost any conversation could end up in an argument over

something simple like what time it was, or the weather outside, or the fact that Grandpa's home was now here with us, not somewhere else. Just as he couldn't let things that irritated him go without challenge, so we had to "put him straight" whenever he said something out of touch with reality. In my viewpoint, he was wrong; I was right. When Grandpa bothered me with his tirades, one solution I found was to leave the room and go somewhere he couldn't see me, where I wouldn't be tempted to answer him. It took a long time for me to realize that defensiveness on my part was not only ineffective but was actually making Grandpa's outbursts last longer. Once I realized that, and looked for other ways of dealing with him, I found some peace.

Meanwhile, our home was about as peaceful as a forest fire. There was a lot of frustration and no seeming end to it, no escape.

In October our little group of camping friends—families who camped together on weekends two or three times each year—planned to go to a place not more than an hour's drive from home. Camping was Milt's favorite escape from the cares and turmoil of city life, and I had come to enjoy it, too. It was pleasant to relax and sit around a campfire in the evening with the quiet of the woods surrounding us. Moreover, camping was a very inexpensive holiday. With Grandpa at home, we were feeling the need for this release and respite more than ever, but how could we make it possible?

The thought occurred to us that maybe Grandpa would also enjoy going out into the woods. Though he had never wanted to join us when he was younger, he did like to be outdoors. Our little camping trailer had a comfortable bed. We happened to have a secondhand wheelchair with a commode attachment. We could take that for a convenient toilet for him. The weather promised to be perfect for October, the fall colors in full bloom. It was worth a try.

The result was less than perfect, to put it mildly. Instead of having a respite from our task, we compounded its difficulty by taking away Grandpa's familiar surroundings. The contest of wills, the unreasonableness, the frustrating tedium of constant demands on our patience, were revealed to all. Nighttime was the worst, culminating in an hour-long episode in which Grandpa, seated on the commode, graphically described to the entire camp-ground exactly what his problem was and how many pieces of toilet paper he needed to take care of it. The experiment was not a total disaster, but it proved so difficult we knew we could never do it again.

At home, food was a constant preoccupation with Grandpa. When he had nothing else to do, he went to the kitchen and opened the refrigerator, taking things out "to taste." If I took these things away from him, he became angry.

"Grandpa, that's margarine. You aren't supposed to eat that." I reached for the bowl in his hand.

"I want that. Whattsa matter, you! Give it to me!"

"Not that, Grandpa; it's no good for you. I'll get you something good. Come and sit down here."

It helped to have a slice of bread with jelly on it or a plate with an early lunch ready to put in front of him to distract him from whatever might irritate him. For me, food became a key to modifying Grandpa's behavior. It seemed to have a calming effect on him.

Food was a pastime for him whether he ate it or not. Sometimes he hid food from the refrigerator in the drawer under the dish towels. Bananas had a special appeal for him, since he could chew them easily. If I left a bunch of them where he could see them, they soon disappeared, either eaten or hidden in various places throughout the house.

Sometimes I would discover, in a seldom-used cupboard, a thoroughly dried, shriveled-up piece of apple. Grandpa also picked up paring knives, teaspoons, and other small items that caught his eye. I became very possessive about my kitchen knives, not because I was concerned that he might hurt himself with them, but because I had my favorite tools and didn't care to conduct a search each time I needed one. I often made the mistake of grabbing things from him if they were things of value. He couldn't understand the reason, but he recognized my anger. "The lady is mad at me," he'd say, or "They steal everything. They don't give me nothing." I found that the best way to get an object away from him was to offer him something else—either something similar in appearance, or at least something likely to interest him.

A number of times, there were special foods prepared which Grandpa could not resist. In fact, as with a child, there was little point in telling him not to take; the delicacy simply had to be put out of sight and out of reach. At Thanksgiving time, Terese, who had taken a foods course the previous year and enjoyed baking, decided that her contribution to our family feast would be two pumpkin pies. She baked them on Wednesday, and that evening we put them in the refrigerator as far back and as inconspicuously as possible.

On Thanksgiving morning, I was up early and working in the kitchen for some time before Grandpa was up. When he awoke he had his usual substantial breakfast: a big bowl of oatmeal followed by coffee and one or two slices of whole wheat bread with jelly. Terese, Cindy, Milt, and I went to church for about an hour, and when we returned Terese found that one of her pies had several spoonfuls gouged out. She was very upset, demanding that we put a lock on the refrigerator door. Milt pondered this puzzle for a while and then went to the basement. About ten minutes later he announced that our problem was solved. He had fastened a shoestring to a silver bell (it had been a gift for our twenty-fifth anniversary) and tied it to the handle of the refrigerator. Voila! Grandpa could still open the refrigerator and get into things, but at least we would know he was doing it. Of course, the bell was neutral—it rang for all of us. Later it got so annoying that Milt replaced the shoestring with a wire hook that could be removed from the door handle with ease when we were using it.

It seemed to me that Grandpa and the rest of us were embroiled in a vicious circle of constant conflict fed by one side or the other, or both. Grandpa had certain pet peeves that he couldn't let go without comment. One was boys with long hair. (It was when the "hippie" look was popular.) At Christmas our sons, Mike and Mart, were home from college for a one-month holiday, and Mart had let his hair grow long. Grandpa would come upon him, seated at the kitchen table, and start in.

"Are you a girl or a boy? You look like a girl."

Hearing him say this made me angry, partially because I knew he had no right to insult my son, but also because I had struggled with the same feelings myself. It was true: Mart's long, wavy hair could have been the envy of many a girl his age.

Mart continued eating his cereal without looking up.

"When are you going to get a haircut?" Grandpa persisted. "Are you lazy? You're no good!"

"Leave me alone, Grandpa. I'm trying to eat my breakfast."

"Eat. That's all you do. You don't do nothing." He shuffled past the table and over to the cupboard, where I was chopping vegetables. He opened the refrigerator door and began reaching inside.

"What would you like, Grandpa? Let me get it for you." I moved in front of him as I spoke.

"I can do it myself," he answered, incensed that I was barring his way. He saw the sharp paring knife I had been using, picked it up, and put it in his pocket. I took an apple from the refrigerator and set it on the table with a plate.

"Here, Grandpa, would you like an apple?"

He turned to sit down, and as he did so I deftly pulled the paring knife from his pocket, giving him a duller one to use.

"Are you a girl or a boy?" he said again to Mart, who was still at the table. "You look like a girl. When are you going to get a haircut?"

"I like my hair the way it is," Mart replied stoically.

"You should get a haircut. You're tall. You could be a policeman!"

"Grandpa, I don't want to be a policeman." There was just a trace of irritation in his voice.

"You're lazy, that's what you are. You're no good."

"Grandpa, that's not true, and you have no right to talk to him that way!" By now my voice betrayed the anger I was trying to suppress. Why did I feel that I had to speak out? Certainly Mart was not a child to be protected from this assault. If my concern was for Mart, it was misdirected in anger at Grandpa. And Grandpa recognized it at once.

"You always stick up for them," he said, as he cut a bite of apple for himself.

Mart picked up his dish, put it in the sink, and left the room.

About this time, Mike wandered into the kitchen and flicked on the overhead lights, since it was a dull day and our kitchen had no window. I don't know whether Grandpa could tell one boy from the other. They were both six feet tall and lanky; the most obvious difference was their hair. While Mart's was shoulder length, wavy, and blond, Mike's was shorter, bushy, and reddish brown. Helping himself to leftovers from the refrigerator, Mike sat down to eat and picked up a magazine to read at the same time.

"Huh! Lights in the daytime! What's the matter, can't you sit over there?" Grandpa pointed to the dining room table by the big window.

"Grandpa, I'd rather sit here to eat my lunch."

"Yeah? Who will pay for it? You don't care!"

"My dad pays for it. It's okay, Grandpa."

"Huh! That's what you think! You're not supposed to read when you eat. My father was strict about that. Either you read, or you eat. Not both."

Mike kept on reading and eating, while Grandpa continued to exclaim. Just listening to it made my stomach churn. I fixed a slice of bread and jelly for Grandpa and then left the room so I wouldn't explode.

I frequently found myself angry with Grandpa, really angry to the point of wishing him harm. On an early morning in January, before our alarm had rung, Terese, who got up early to catch the school bus, came to our bedroom door and called, "Mom, where's the lunch meat? Are we out of it?" I knew I had just bought some. I got out of bed and went down to look, wondering to myself why other people in the house became blind when it came to finding things. I opened the refrigerator and looked: on the shelf, in the drawers, in the door compartment. The package of lunch meat should have been there, but it was not.

Later I was making Cindy's breakfast when Grandpa got up. He came from his bedroom into the kitchen carrying the package of lunch meat that should have been in the refrigerator. "I found this in there," he said. "I don't know what it is."

Taking it from him, I was suddenly filled with anger. I could feel the blood rushing into my head. My arms and legs were shaking.

"You shouldn't take things like that, Grandpa!" I scowled at him. "Now it's spoiled; wasted! Meat must be kept in the refrigerator. There's plenty of food here for you. You don't have to take it and hide it!"

He didn't say a word, just walked away, but I knew he felt hurt by my outburst. I felt a little remorseful because I knew he didn't know what he was doing, but I still felt angry as I threw the package into the garbage.

"I wish I had the nerve to feed it to him," I thought. "If he got sick I wouldn't care." I began making his oatmeal, and soon he was back in the kitchen. I held out to him the cup with his false teeth. He took the denture and placed it in his mouth. "Now go get your shirt, Grandpa, and put it on." He left again, and I noticed that I was still shaking with anger. I didn't want to talk to him. He came back to eat, and I gave him his oatmeal. I made myself a cup of coffee, but instead of sitting down with him I stood at the cupboard with my back to him. "Why am I so angry?" I asked myself. I began to feel more calm.

Later, after Terese, Milt, and Cindy had gone, Grandpa stood at the window exclaiming about the snow. He was worried that there was so much of it, and it was still coming down. "There were times, I remember," he said, "when there was so much snow that the streetcars all stopped and no one could go anywhere. . . . What should I do about food?"

"I'll take care of it, don't worry," I answered. He asked how much bread we had, so I showed him the half-empty loaf. He wanted to go and buy some. I said, "No, I'm going. You stay here." I was still angry with him. It would be good to go outside and get away from him.

We went to the door and looked out. The snow was deeper than I thought—five inches already. I would have to shovel the driveway before taking the car out. I put on my ski jacket and my boots. Grandpa wanted to go out to "clean up the snow" too, but he had only cloth shoes on. I got out Milt's boots, put them on him, and helped him with his coat and hat. Then I went to the garage for shovels and gave him the lighter one. As I started shoveling, I felt good that I could do some physical work. I threw each shovelful of snow as hard as I could. I asked myself whether I was deliberately persisting in feeling angry with Grandpa, even enjoying it. He came up behind me and started shoveling, blocking my way. Again I was irritated. I told him to work under the carport where the snow was less deep, but he insisted on "helping" me. I felt like pushing him. Again I was amazed that I was still feeling so angry about a package of lunch meat. I showed him that he could shovel forward along the edge of the drive and I could shovel the rest of the width, so he wouldn't be in my way. We worked together for some time. Gradually I realized that I did want to be angry; I was deliberately choosing it. What was missing was prayer; a real desire on my part to forgive Grandpa and tolerate his shortcomings. I was closing myself off from the spirit of God within me, which prompted me to accept Grandpa just the way he was. Now I could see that what had happened was just another opportunity. I could have taken it either way. It was a choice. Next time, I hoped to make a better choice.

We finished clearing the driveway and drove to the grocery store together for bread, lunch meat, and a few other items. It stopped snowing, and when we returned the whole landscape was a crystal paradise gleaming in the sunshine.

Milt did not fully agree with the way I gave Grandpa bread and jelly all the time. He became concerned that Grandpa was putting on too much weight. He envisioned the possibility of having to lift him at some future time, while to me this was so far in the future that it was unimportant. Grandpa had lost considerable weight during his illness and hospitalization. He had gained it back rapidly and was still gaining, though not as fast. Terese joined with Milt in conspiring to keep Grandpa's weight under control. They would either refuse him snacks or give him something low in calories:

"No fancy stuff. Just give me bread. I'm hungry."

"You already had your breakfast at eight o'clock."

"No, I didn't have anything to eat. I'm hungry. Give me bread."

"Grandpa, eat this grapefruit. It's good," Terese tried to persuade him.

"No, I don't want it. It won't fill me up. I'm weak." As if to prove this, he dropped his arms heavily to his sides, slumped forward in his chair, and hung his head loosely. He was very convincing!

"But you need vitamins, too. You've had enough bread today."

"If you won't give me bread I won't eat nothing. No." Then he would sulk until someone would relent and give him what he wanted.

We constantly felt ourselves in a "catch-22" situation with Grandpa. He wanted conversation, yet it seemed that whatever we said to him, it was the wrong thing. We found it hard to agree with him, even in simple matters, because we wanted him to face the truth of what day it was, or what time it was, or where he was, or whose object he had in his hand.

There was no way to make him face the truth. Any amount of disagreement led to a long diatribe. One day he and I were looking at his photo album. He saw the picture of himself and his wife together with several of our children on the occasion of Pat's first Holy Communion some thirteen years before. He made the comment, "I like children. I don't know who they are, but I take care of them."

Obviously this was not true, so I tried to straighten his thoughts out: "Those are your grandchildren. You were not taking care of them, they were just visiting you that day."

This innocent statement of mine set off a chain reaction of repetitive statements: "I take care of the children. I don't let them get hurt. I don't know where the parents are, but I take care of them."

He repeated the same refrain over and over as I tried to distract him by directing his attention to other pictures. Toward the back of the book, we came to a picture of Milt as a child of eight or so, standing on a small ladder which was against a tree. Grandpa saw this and again began repeating "I don't know who the parents are, but I take care of the children. He wants a big ladder, but I tell him, 'No, not until you get big.' I don't want to be responsible. Children are reckless, they can fall. I don't want them to get hurt."

My efforts to point out who this child was and that he was the parent of this child were fruitless. He denied it. Milt walked in at that point, and I said, "Here he is, the boy in the picture. That's your son, Milt."

But he said, "No, I don't know who that is," and we closed the book. It was primarily Milt and I who had this difficulty in communication with him. Mike and Terese were able to talk with him much more successfully. Somehow we were reluctant to learn from them.

Grandpa's claim that he cared for children was not borne out by his relationship with Cindy. There seemed to be a pecking order in our house, and if Grandpa was the frequent recipient of criticism, he, in turn, could usually pick on Cindy, and vice versa.

Customarily, Cindy was asked to clear, wipe, and set the kitchen table in preparation for the evening meal. On one occasion, she picked up Grandpa's glasses, which he often left there, and handed them to him, saying, "Grandpa, you're supposed to keep these in your bedroom. They don't belong in the kitchen. Put them away, please."

"I always keep the glasses here. That's where they belong. What do you mean, I have to stay there? What, are you the boss? She tells me I don't belong here."

I was drawn into it: "Grandpa, that's not true. She said your glasses don't belong here. You do belong here. This is your home too."

"They tell me I can't be here. I don't belong here."

"That's not what she said, Grandpa. You can be wherever you want. You do belong here." Here I was again, settling squabbles between "siblings."

Again, the doorbell rang on a Saturday afternoon. Cindy's friend Krista had brought some jacks and wanted to play. The two girls, both blond and wiry, sat on the floor in the family room, gradually becoming a little boisterous and giggly as they tossed the small ball and bounded after it.

"Is that the way you behave in the house?" Grandpa demanded, standing over them menacingly.

Cindy looked apologetically toward Krista and answered, "We're just playing jacks, Grandpa."

"My parents were strict. No balls in the house. You should play outside."

"Grandpa is mean sometimes," Cindy explained in a quiet voice.

"I know. My grandmother is mean lots of times, too."

"We could go up in my room and play."

"Okay."

They gathered their things and scooted around him and up the stairs. Later they came to the kitchen for a snack. Grandpa had just finished having some bread and jelly and a cup of coffee. Cindy took some fruit from the refrigerator, and the two girls scurried into the family room. Grandpa followed after them.

"Go outside!" he said gruffly. "Go on!"

I heard what was going on as I came up from the basement. "Grandpa, you have no business telling Cindy and her friend to go outside!" I felt hurt and embarrassed for Cindy. I wanted to punish him in some way. Grabbing him by the arms, I turned him firmly back toward the kitchen. "I'm sorry Cindy, Krista. Just don't pay any attention to him." But they went outside anyway, and I couldn't blame Krista if she chose not to come back very soon. It was hard to have fun with Grandpa around.

One day in February, Milt reported that Mrs. Rossi, one of his teachers, was looking for someone to keep her little dog during her family's spring vacation in Florida. She happened to know that our Cindy loved dogs, and wondered if she could pay Cindy to take care of Maggie for that week.

Cindy's eyes sparkled. She would almost pay for the privilege!

"What about Grandpa?" I asked. I knew he didn't like dogs.

"Well, it's only for one week," Milt said.

"Please, Mom, can I? It won't be any trouble. I promise!"

I felt that Cindy, aged eleven now, was getting the "short end of the stick," so to speak, in this project of caring for Grandpa, so I didn't have the heart to say no. Instead I suggested a trial period. Maggie came to stay overnight that Friday, and I must admit that she won me over. The answer had to be yes.

Maggie was a little black poodle, a curly haired ball of fluff. I had always thought poodles were nervous dogs that barked all the time; I had seen some that acted that way. Maggie, however, was the sweetest-tempered dog I had ever seen. She didn't bark at all until she had been with us for two or three days, and then it was more a comment than a bark.

Maggie followed Cindy around, or sat and watched what was going on, or slept, or begged food from Cindy or the rest of us by standing quietly and looking up with big, brown, hungry-looking eyes. We found that Maggie had a taste for lasagna, bananas, liver sausage, apples, yogurt, jelly beans, and chocolate Easter eggs. She didn't much care for plain hamburger, cheese, or peanut butter (except on toast). She liked to play rough with Cindy but was careful not to bite too hard, and when Cindy would say, "Stop!" she would stop.

Maggie was never insistent on being taken outside. One morning Cindy slept until nine-thirty or so, and Maggie didn't seem to mind at all.

In short, Maggie was a delight to have around, and certainly didn't cause any trouble. Except that Grandpa didn't like her. In fact, he "barked" and hollered and carried on just about every time he saw her. Cindy tried to keep them in different rooms, but that was difficult to do.

Grandpa thought of dogs as being "outside" animals. They should not be in the house. Furthermore, the only reason for a dog's existence was to be a watchdog. Maggie was obviously not a watchdog; therefore she had no possible use whatsoever, according to him.

From the way Grandpa talked, it seemed that he was sure Maggie was not house-trained and would leave a trail behind her for him to clean up!

Grandpa would sometimes smile when he saw Cindy playing with Maggie, but not for long. The next thing we would hear was "Get that hound out of here! Throw it out!"

One morning Maggie came downstairs before Cindy was up. She may have wanted to go out, because the small black poodle was sitting quietly by the front door when Grandpa saw her. I could hardly believe my ears when he began saying, "C'mon, c'mon," to her in a sugary sweet voice.

The next minute Terese, who happened to be coming down the stairs and saw them, ran over to the door shouting, "Grandpa, don't do that!" He had picked up poor Maggie by her collar and was about to throw her out the door!

Grandpa showed signs of being jealous of Maggie. When Cindy fed something to Maggie, Grandpa said, "Humph, the dog gets food, but what about me?" Of course, Maggie was getting a lot of attention—something Grandpa couldn't get enough of.

Other than jealousy, we could see no reason for Grandpa's deep-seated hatred of Maggie. Even the fact that she was not a watchdog didn't seem to account for his violent reaction. Terese tried to remind him that he had once had two birds for pets, and they certainly hadn't been useful either, but he didn't remember them anymore; he said she was lying.

I guess we will never know what caused all that hostility to pour out on one small, black, well-behaved poodle. Fortunately, it didn't seem to hurt Maggie in the least.

This first year of caring for Grandpa was the most difficult one. There were so many adjustments to be made—staying home instead of going out, enduring his angry outbursts and constant demands. For his part, Grandpa had to put up with new surroundings, our lack of time for him, our need for control. Tempers flared on both sides.

While the day-to-day response to Grandpa's ups and downs went on, I became more and more aware that I was getting tired of taking on the major role in this project. During the twenty-five years of my marriage, my customary way of coping with any perceived unfairness in the allotment of chores was one of quiet acquiescence, with undercurrents of resentment that flared up in sudden bursts of anger at the children, periods of "silent treatment" for Milt, or both. I could see my anger erupting at Grandpa. I sometimes had a very short fuse and didn't care to quench it. I knew myself well enough to know that I was in danger of sinking into a mire of resentment over this change in my life, but I was determined not to permit this to happen.

I began to look for ways in which I could continue to grow

and be nurtured at home. I knew I would need to set aside some time just for myself.

First, there was exercise. I had taken two or three classes in yoga and had enjoyed the stretching, bending, and flexing of muscles and joints at a slow, easy, relaxing pace. Now I decided I knew enough to continue on my own, at home. In the morning, when Milt got up, I began my yoga warm-ups before even getting out of bed. Then, standing beside the bed, I proceeded with the "sun greeting," an exercise of almost every muscle and joint in the body. When done slowly, through two routines, this takes about five minutes. I added other specific exercises that I thought my body particularly needed—movements of arms, shoulders, neck, spine, hips, and knees. The routine of one exercise after another, in set sequence, carried me along. The entire routine took twenty or twenty-five minutes. It felt very good. I let everyone else take care of their breakfast needs and Grandpa too, if necessary, while I exercised. I was "busy."

After Milt left for work and the house was quiet, I would make sure that Grandpa had his breakfast in front of him, and I would take the next half hour to forty-five minutes just to sit quietly, pray, read the Bible, and meditate. I had never read the Bible on my own before, but it happened that because of our involvement in Young Life (an ecumenical Christian ministry to high-school students), we had received in the mail a sample copy of a Bible study guide, a monthly publication called *Ventures*. I began using it and subsequently subscribed to it because it satisfied my need for a home program of Bible study and prayer. Many times Grandpa would interrupt my quiet time, but I refused to let that bother me: I expected it. When it didn't happen, I was thankful.

Taking this time for myself in the morning meant that I had even less time during the day to accomplish whatever tasks I had to do—besides spending time with Grandpa. But I didn't care. There were days when I accomplished very little. The house didn't get cleaned as often or as thoroughly; the bedding no longer got changed every week. Things that had to be done, like laundry, grocery shopping, and meal preparations, were done as needed. The house did not fall apart from neglect.

Of all of the family, I spent the most time with Grandpa, and naturally I learned better than anyone else how to manage him. I could ascertain his moods—when he was content to be left alone, when he needed something to do, when he needed company or cheering up. I made it my project to be aware of all these things and to respond to them when necessary but to continue my own pursuits in the meantime.

Other members of the family—particularly Milt—were impressed with the way I could get Grandpa to do what I wanted him to do. If we were going somewhere in the car, for example, I had certain words that I always used, and I spoke them slowly, loud enough for him to hear: "Grandpa, I have to go someplace, and I want you to come with me."

I might have to repeat once or twice until he could understand. The same words could be used when we wanted Grandpa to go upstairs to take a shower, or when I thought he might need a trip to the bathroom.

Milt, on the other hand, thought Grandpa should respond at once to his command. Grandpa was no longer a father figure to Milt. Now he was dependent, like a child; therefore he should obey like a child. Milt's patience was in short supply when Grandpa refused or was reluctant to comply. They ended up yelling at one another.

It was obvious to me that my way worked better. I would have liked Milt to watch how I managed Grandpa and to learn how to do it himself. Instead, he let me do it. I became the expert caretaker.

Milt and I had a solid, nurturing relationship, but there were areas where I was less assertive than I needed to be, and where Milt was less sensitive than he could have been. Having his dad was at first my responsibility because I was home, I was capable, I was the expert. Day and night, whether Milt was home or not, I was the one who heard Grandpa's call first and who got up to answer it first.

There was one area that Milt made his special concern: showering Grandpa. Personal cleanliness was something Grandpa had definite ideas about. All he needed or wanted was a small towel, a washcloth, and a comb. He washed his face and hands every morning and combed his hair. Living on the first floor of our home was convenient for him, but there was only a half bath at that level; the tub and shower were on the second floor. We began a weekly routine of inviting Grandpa upstairs to have his shower on a weekend evening when it was convenient for Milt. Grandpa's cooperation was necessary, so if he refused or made a fuss, we'd wait until the next night. It was a private time for Milt and his dad. They would go upstairs together, Grandpa following, and Milt would explain that Grandpa was going to have a shower.

"What for? I'm not dirty," Grandpa would insist.

"Well, everybody takes baths, Dad. We sweat, we need to wash."

Usually Grandpa would comply. Milt had to overcome feelings of embarrassment at seeing his father nude, but Grandpa didn't make any issue about that. He washed himself thoroughly and seemed to take pride in doing it. Milt would stand by in his shorts, lathering up the washcloth, washing Grandpa's back, and then giving him a shampoo. Grandpa's hair was gray and soft, with a little wave to it, and it looked especially nice after being washed. His only complaint about showering was that he had to stand too long, so Milt found an old metal stool in the basement (a relic of Grandpa's) that was just the right height for him to sit on while Milt washed his hair.

Meanwhile, I would pick up Grandpa's soiled clothes and lay out his clean ones. He would dress himself, with a little help from Milt where needed, and come downstairs in good spirits.

One day Grandpa had been arranging his wood scraps in his bedroom workshop, and I could tell by his language that there was some sort of problem or frustration. I was writing a letter and didn't go to inquire about it.

He came into the family room, used the bathroom, and then stopped to say, "If I had money, I might be able to get some food."

Instead of just getting him something to eat, I thought I would quiz him a little bit, so I asked, "What would you do if you had money in your pocket?"

"Well, I'd go out and go to some stores."

"Did you do that lately?"

"No."

"When did you eat last?"

"Yesterday."

"Where did you get the food then?"

"Well, I guess I went there and asked those people for some-thing. I used to get money, but now it goes to that organization and I don't get nothing."

"What place is this, where you are?"

"Well, it's—they let me sleep here sometimes."

"What kind of place is it? What do you do here?"

"Well, I help the people. That's that organization. Oh, the hell with you and your questions! I don't want to bother with you. Get out of here!" He walked off, got his pipe, and had a smoke.

There were many hours of the day when Grandpa needed verbal communication and stimulation. I liked to use his photo album, which I had put together for him and Babi before she died. It provided good conversation-starters. He remembered some of the people in the pictures and would talk about them. He didn't know that the children were his grandchildren, but the pictures of his home and garden, his wife and friends, prompted deeper memories that were still intact. His favorites were pictures of himself, standing proudly in front of his garden, or on his back porch with his many pots of geraniums. He was happy to talk about these to anyone who would sit down with him and look at the album. It was a natural way to converse with Grandpa, and it was more interesting than his usual monologue.

Another idea I tried was getting Grandpa to read to me. I found a couple of old Bohemian books among his things, so I asked him to translate for me. This he did in a phrase-by-phrase, halting fashion that hardly made sense. But we passed some time trying. Terese came home from the library with some *Reader's Digest* magazines in large print for him. I thought it was a good idea because this had been his favorite magazine, but now it failed to capture his interest.

I was determined to continue with as many activities as I could during the day, especially grocery shopping, and taking Grandpa with me in the car became a frequent necessity. I shopped several days each week, so that it never tired Grandpa too much. Many times when I was ready to leave for the store he would refuse.

I would just wait awhile, perhaps give him a bit to eat, and then try again. Going to the grocery store was particularly good for him because he was with people and he was helping me: he pushed the cart. Holding on to it even steadied his walk. When he saw small children in the store, he often stopped to say a few words to them, and he obviously enjoyed it when they responded with a smile or an answer.

Three or four times a month, I took Grandpa with me to Resource: for Affirmative Living (RE:AL), where I worked as a volunteer. RE:AL was a nonprofit organization that served our community by providing classes in crafts, exercise, parenting skills, and any topics of current interest primarily to women. I had joined the group seven years earlier, and as my enjoyment of this outlet for my energy grew, so did my commitment to it. I helped in the office and with the newsletter. Eventually I was asked to take on the jobs of newsletter editor and mailing coordinator, which automatically made me a member of the board of directors, a stimulating group of active women. I felt affirmed and challenged as a person apart from my husband and children for the first time in my life. Milt was very supportive of this activity, but we both understood that this was in addition to my traditional work of maintaining our home and family.

Besides the RE:AL newsletter, there was a program booklet that had to be collated, stapled, and mailed out in fall, winter, and spring. A group of six or seven women—or as many as I could muster—would gather to help. They became used to seeing Grandpa, and they made a point of speaking to him and being friendly. Two of the women in particular would go out of their way to greet him warmly with spontaneous hugs (something I could not feel comfortable enough to do) and to pay attention to him frequently as we worked. Grandpa responded beautifully and made conversation as best he could.

We would sit at tables in the largest room of the church basement where the RE:AL Center was located, to fold and staple our material. I would put Grandpa next to me and keep him supplied with some sheets of paper to fold. He was able to do simple operations following directions. I would give him a stack of papers and ask him to fold them in half; and he would be meticulous about putting the corners together. As soon as he finished, I would give him more. When I saw that he was tired, I'd get him some coffee or cookies so he wouldn't start insisting on going home.

One of the most special occasions in RE:AL's year was the spring luncheon. It was a time for all the volunteers and participants to celebrate together the good feelings that had been cultivated during the year. Grandpa's coming had prevented me from participating in daytime classes, but I had continued serving on the board, chairing the mailing committee, and editing the newsletter, the latter of which I was able to do at home.

In the spring of 1979, one year after Grandpa had come to live with us, I struggled with the question of how I could attend the spring luncheon. At this point I had exhausted the sitters who had answered my ad in the newspaper and any "baby-sitters" on my list. I relied on Milt and, occasionally, the children (mainly Terese and Cindy) to stay with Grandpa when I really wanted to go somewhere. The luncheon, was, of course, in the afternoon, when Terese and Cindy were in school and Milt was at work. My only hope was Mike, who was home from college for the summer. He did not yet have a summer job lined up, but he didn't seem to be too worried about it. I had already asked him about the luncheon once, without getting a definite answer, so I brought it to his attention a second time.

"Mike, remember I asked you if you could stay with Grandpa next Friday afternoon? Could you? RE:AL is having their spring luncheon from twelve-thirty till about three-thirty and I'd really like to go."

"Well, I don't know. I might be busy."

"Do you have some definite plans?"

"No, not now, but I might."

"Well, if it's not something definite, I wish you'd consider staying with Grandpa for me. This luncheon is only once a year, and I need to buy my ticket by Tuesday. When could you let me know?"

"I don't know; I'd have to think about it."

"Okay. . . ." I couldn't understand his reluctance. Of all the children, Mike was the one who really cared about Grandpa and spent time talking with him, teasing him, making him laugh. He really loved Grandpa. I wasn't so sure about his feelings for me.

The next day I broached the topic again. "Mike, I don't want to pester you about it, but I really have to know if I can go to that luncheon or not. Do you think you could stay with Grandpa on Friday? It's only for three hours or so."

"I don't know what I'm going to be doing on Friday."

"This is really important to me, Mike. You haven't got that much to do right now; what does it matter?"

"It does matter. I want to do what I want to do, that's all."

"Well, it seems to me that you could do this special favor for me. You don't mind being with Grandpa, do you?"

He was silent for a long moment. "No, I guess I can do it. Yeah, I'll stay with him."

"Okay, thanks, Mike. I appreciate it." I bought my ticket and looked forward to enjoying a carefree afternoon with my friends.

Friday came, and it was a beautiful day. Grandpa sat outside smoking his pipe in the warm sunshine. He cut several pieces of wood and then rested, enjoying another smoke. "This is my friend," he said, referring to his pipe. "I used to smoke, what do you call those . . . [cigarettes—he couldn't think of the word], but this is the best." Grandpa was having a good day, too.

Suddenly Mike said, "Mom, could you be home by two-thirty? I have to go to the YMCA for a job interview."

I was stunned. I couldn't believe Mike would do this to me. "Mike, you said you would stay with Grandpa. Why did you make an appointment with someone else?" I could feel myself flushing with anger, my voice becoming higher, louder, as I spoke.

"Well, I just thought you could come home earlier."

"You could have asked me first! You have no consideration for me! All you care about is yourself!" Now I was out of control, but I didn't care.

"That's why I don't like to say ahead of time that I'll stay at home, because there might be something that I need to do."

"You had all week long to set up your interview. You just didn't do it because you didn't care. You men are all alike. It's 'Me First,' and it's probably my fault for raising you to be a chauvinist!"

"What about Mart? Is he a chauvinist too?"

"Yes, he is, and he's probably worse than you are. He's never available at all, and that's the way he likes it. Well, I have to get dressed now. Sure, I can come home earlier. I'll be here at two-thirty." I spat out the words.

The RE:AL luncheon was marvelous. The committee had gone all-out to make it an occasion of beauty, elegance, and friendship. The buffet table gleamed with a centerpiece of molded ice and flowers created by the chairperson, who was also the caterer of the food. The people involved in this group were incredible. They didn't stop at just giving; they gave from their hearts.

The lunch got started a little late, and the program started later, but no one seemed to care—except me, because I was keeping an eye on my watch. To foster camaraderie, the theme of the luncheon was sharing from our past. Each of us was asked to tell where she was born and something about her childhood. The conversation at my table revealed that some of us had originated in small Illinois towns very close to one another and had attended schools that competed in sports. Except for age differences, we might have cheered at the same basketball games! It was a fun discovery.

The entertainment went on, and I cherished every moment. Finally it was time for me to leave, and I struggled with a feeling of incompleteness due to more than simply missing some of the program.

I drove home, parked the car in the driveway, and went inside. Grandpa was sitting in his usual chair in the family room, talking to himself. Mike was sitting on the sofa in the living room, reading.

"I'm not going to the 'Y' after all," he said. "You didn't have to come home early."

"Didn't have to come home!" I almost screamed at him. "Why didn't you tell me? Why didn't you call me at the Center?" I was so angry and hurt that I dashed up the stairs to my bedroom and into the bathroom, closing the door behind me. I sat for a moment, letting the realization of what had happened come over me. Was I crazy? Did I make this up? Did Mike first tell me he'd be here, then that I should be home early, then change his plans again and not tell me? Suddenly it was too much. I began to cry as I have seldom cried, wailing like a child, sobbing convulsively, tears streaming down my face. For a few moments I just let go, not caring about anything. Then I heard Terese's voice at the door. She had come home early from school.

"Mom, what's the matter?" she asked in a concerned tone of voice.

"Nothing. Ask Mike," I answered, now beginning to feel embarrassed at being caught. I wiped my eyes, blew my nose, dashed cold water on my face, and patted it dry with a towel. "Well, I've had my afternoon off; now it's back to work again." I said to myself. "Let's see. What was I going to make for supper?"

5 · The Second Year

The first section of this chapter was written by Terese when she was sixteen. She became very close to her grandfather and delighted in his company. She presents her own perspective of those first two years.

TERESE'S STORY: GRANDPA, THE STROLLING MUSICIAN

When I was a child, Grandpa frightened me. He has been hard of hearing for as long as I can remember. I could never really speak with him because I couldn't talk loud enough, or was afraid to. We used to go over to his house once in a while. It smelled . . . different. Like an old person's house. It was rather cluttered. He used to have two birds. He built a large cage for them in the kitchen, but he also let them fly around the outside of the cage. He had cut-up cereal boxes on the curtain-tops, where they perched. In my mind I have a memory of him rubbing some ointment on a poor, sick bird; I felt sorry for it, crumpled in his hand.

Once, when I was about seven, I stood looking at the figurines in a glass case in his dining room, and he said I could pick out any one and keep it for myself. I picked out a fancy painted egg. It was a real egg, and it was all covered with very tiny brown painted lines in a certain pattern. It rattled when you shook it gently. My mom said the yolk was all hard and dry inside. I had it in my room for a long time, until it broke.

When we used to go and visit Grandpa, he always

sent home some coins for us to divide into six piles, one for each grandchild. He called it "chicken-feed."

One time when he came to our house on Christmas Eve, I remember that I was impatient to open presents. Grandpa wanted to watch a sort of Western program on TV first. I think it was on until six o'clock. So the whole family had to wait. I remember feeling angry at him for keeping me waiting.

When Grandpa came here to stay, it was different. I was much older, and he was weak from being sick. We had to get reacquainted with each other. I liked to ask him questions about when he was young, and I liked him to teach me to say words in Bohemian.

Grandpa is very dependent on us. He's like a child. One day when he was still new here I was "senior-sitting" him because he can't stay alone. (Cindy and I started out calling it baby-sitting, but we changed it to senior-sitting because Grandpa is a senior citizen.) I was very busy with my own things upstairs when I heard him messing around in the kitchen. I crept down and watched him from the stairs. He was mumbling while going through the refrigerator. I was surprised that he would open our refrigerator because I felt he had no right to do that.

I knew that Grandpa enjoyed music. When he was young, he played the concertina and must have been very good at it because he played at dances. Also, ever since I can remember, whenever Grandpa was offered some beer or wine, he always said, "If I drink this, I'll sing!" He said it to make a joke. But I had never heard him sing. Some time ago I was playing "Happy Birthday" on the piano, and I didn't know that Grandpa was in a chair right behind me. He started humming along with my music. He told me that he remembered that song. He sang the melody all the way through by himself. I was shocked! (When Grandpa sings, he usually doesn't sing words, just na-na-na, or dee-dee-dee, or dah-dah-dah.) Besides that once, though, he didn't sing any more.

Then, last Christmas, which was five months ago, I was playing "Silent Night" on the piano, and he heard me and sang along. On a piece of paper, I wrote the words to it. He knew the melody, so he could transfer it to the words. It was great! He got a lot of encouragement from all of us to keep singing it. I also wrote down the words to "Happy Birthday" for him.

I tried to think of what other song Grandpa might remember. "Jingle Bells," perhaps? I played it for him on the piano, and he knew it! So I wrote out the words to that one, too. During that time when we encouraged him to sing, he was coming up with other songs he remembered from long ago, some American, some Bohemian. Now he sings all the time! His repertoire has really increased:

"Let Me Call You Sweetheart"
"Kill Another Dutchman"
"Butchke Ya Boshya" (My own phonetic spelling!)
"Shla Na Ninka Dozali"
"Jingle Bells"
"Me Lu Esha, Boshuecsh Mom Kay Lad"
"Silent Night" (by request only)
"Cheeri Biri Bin"

His singing is great. Whenever Grandpa feels down and thinks he's no good because he can't work, I always ask him to sing: "spee-vay" (in Bohemian). I tell him that is the way he can help us. So he does, and it cheers him up. It makes us and him happy!

That's why I like to joke about him being a strolling musician. He just shuffles around the house singing.

When Grandpa becomes very angry, he occasionally runs away. He just goes outside and keeps walking. The first time this happened was the summer when he first came. I was alone with him. He became very angry and told me he was walking home. When I told him that his home in Cicero was twelve miles away, he was not a bit discouraged. He walked down our driveway and promptly turned left. I ran outside and walked with him—in my socks. All the while he walked, I tried to talk him into turning around and going home. "No!" was his firm answer. When he approached the corner, he turned right and crossed the street. He said things like, "Where's a policeman? I'm going to have him take me to jail. At least I'll get food there!" He was sure about that!

We walked the next two blocks slowly. Grandpa doesn't ever walk much. Our neighbor, Mr. Micek, saw us and thought I might be having trouble. He parked his car ahead of us, got out, and said, "Hi, Frank! How are you?" Grandpa does not know this man, but he said hello. Mr. Micek asked Grandpa if he needed a ride home. Grandpa accepted, so we both got in the car, and Mr. Micek drove us right back to where we walked from. Grandpa was angry that Mr. Micek had brought him back to the place he was before. I can't remember what happened next. (This was long ago.)

Another time, Grandpa tried to run away when Cindy and I were senior-sitting him one night during the winter. We were both busy with homework and didn't have time to talk with him. He became angry and announced that he was going home. Cindy double-locked our door so that it could not be opened without a key. The fact that Grandpa couldn't get the door open made him very upset. His eyes flared! He ordered us to open the door, but we just couldn't. We didn't have time to walk with him; we also didn't want him outside on a dark winter night.

On both sides of our front door are panels of glass. Grandpa stood there and banged on them. He shouted, "I won't stop until you open!" Then he got a piece of hard plastic and scraped it back and forth on the glass, making a terrible sound.

I was getting fed up with him. I set the kitchen timer for five minutes and went to talk with him. At first the only word he would shout was, "Open!" Gradually he calmed down. He sat, and we talked. (I had to stretch the five minutes to twenty.) Soon he was very grateful;

he held my hand and stroked it. He said, "You're so good!" This clearly showed me that when Grandpa is upset, 99% of the time it is because he need some loving attention.

Grandpa's happiness is the best thing about him. I love it! He says he likes to "have a little fun." He teases, jokes, and laughs. I think he's the most fun of anyone in our family.

One day Grandpa was sitting down with his hands crossed, and he was singing. I asked him if he could "do this," and I twiddled my thumbs. Then he tried it, going very slowly for a moment. Then he broke into a super-fast twiddle! We laughed hard. He said, "I surprised you, didn't I? When I was young I used to do this while I waited for the bus I took to work."

I was washing the supper dishes and had a sink full of sudsy water. I got a huge handful of the fluffy bubbles and walked over to Grandpa. He was sitting with my dad, a few feet away from the sink. "Look!" I said.

"Mmm! My!" he said.

I moved my hand of bubbles, teasing him, next to his hand.

"Uh uh," he said, meaning "no."

"Come on." I coaxed him.

He shook hands with me. We were all squishy with suds. With his hand all wet and frothy, he motioned to my dad and asked, "Would you like to shake, young man?"

Of course my dad refused. We laughed real hard at that! I love it when Grandpa plays with me and does things that a "proper adult" wouldn't do! He smiled some more; then broke into a chorus of "Jingle Bells"!

The Jedachek (that's the Bohemian word for Grandpa that I like to call him sometimes) was fishing around in his bedroom closet and came out with a black cane we got for him when he returned from the hospital. He shoved it in my hands and said, "When you're with your friends, you walk with this and they'll think you're something special."

I told him, "Grandpa, I don't know how to walk with a cane!" Canes are so tippy that I don't understand how they could help anyone walk.

He took it and, without hesitating, started to proudly and slowly strut around the room, swinging the cane like a distinguished man. He even tipped his head to the left and looked up in the air, like a stuck-up person.

I loved it! For the next ten minutes we laughed and practiced walking like a "rich man"!

Grandpa was a great actor. His imagination took over whenever he didn't have the facts. He had a soreness in his left arm and shoulder. The doctor said it was bursitis. When it bothered him a lot, he told us that two men hit him in the arm. He would groan like it was happening all over again. When he woke up in the morning, he would hold his arm stiffly down at his side and walk haltingly, bending way over. If I went over to him, he jerked suddenly, as if I had done something to make it sore, even if I hadn't touched him at all. My mom would have a heating pad ready for him, but usually he didn't want it. Sometimes she gave him an aspirin. After he started eating, I guess the arm would feel better, because he would forget all about it. Later he stretched the story. It became four men who hit him with an iron bar! We would all laugh to ourselves about it, but Grandpa was serious. He was just trying to tell us how much pain he had. Occasionally he would tell the story to strangers, and that was embarrassing. They might think that we did it!

Sometimes Grandpa was very weak. Maybe he was hungry or just tired. He would tell us that he felt weak, but that wasn't enough. He acted it out. He would put on the expression of someone half asleep, hanging his head down and leaning over like he was about to fall. He could even do it when he was standing up! He made me think he was going to die! As soon as he had something to eat or got into a better mood, though, he was as strong as ever. We joked that Grandpa should win an Academy Award.

Another thing that is great about Grandpa is his lovableness. I put my arm around him, shake his hand, rub his back. He's so easy to love because he holds no grudge. He has a terrible memory; he can't remember from one minute to another. If we get into a fight, ten minutes later we can be pals.

Once when Mart was home, he, Cindy, Grandpa, and I were all sitting around the kitchen table singing together and moving our hands and arms like an orchestra conductor does. Grandpa looked me in the eye while we sang, and that was the happiest I've ever seen him. His eyes literally sparkled! I was very happy from just looking at him.

I really like to give Grandpa a challenge by playing catch with him. He usually insists that he isn't able to catch or throw a tennis ball. While he is sitting down I take aim, and he tries to focus on the ball. He looks real funny; he moves his eyebrows up and down. Then I toss it gently, and he jerks his body and uses every bit of effort he has to catch it.

He throws it back underhand, and if he throws it a little bit off, he moves his hand in exasperation and says, "Shucks!"

I've been trying to learn to juggle, and when I juggle outside I like to have Grandpa around to fetch balls. He walks around and picks them up without being asked. A couple of days ago I made a record—I juggled 233 times without stopping. While I was doing it, Grandpa said, "Moy, moy," (he says "my" but puts an "o" sound in it) and "My, you must be making a record!"

Grandpa loves to shake hands, and so do I. He squeezes my hand as hard as he can until I scream, "Stop!" But sometimes I squeeze back almost as hard. He tells me, "My, you're strong! You've got a grip!" and I tell him, "So do you." We love it. Sometimes when we shake hands we aren't so rough, and he moves my hand to the beat of the song he's singing. I like to do the same, but I surprise him and move his hand in a sporadic way. He doesn't know quite what to expect.

During the wintertime, every time I shake his hand he says, "My, you have warm hands! Mine are cold, huh?" and I say, "Yeah." Then he says, "Say, what do you drink?" and I tell him, "Whiskey!" Then he laughs real hard, gives me a questioning look, and says "No?"

On Holy Thursday, before Easter Sunday, Mom, Dad, Cindy, Grandpa, and I went to an "agape" dinner (pot-luck) at our church, and to Mass afterward. I hate it when we have to bring Grandpa. It's embarrassing! He doesn't understand that he's supposed to shut up; he's just like a little kid. He hates it when I put my hand over his mouth to shush him, or put my finger to my mouth; he wants an answer to his question or statement.

So, there we are in a quiet church, and he says, very loud, "Next time, I'll stay home!" Ten heads turn to look at him. Then he yawns very loudly and says, "Ya—ya," with a sigh.

During the "kiss of peace," Grandpa shook a few hands, which he loves to do. He was happy, so he hummed his "Jingle Bells." It's a good thing that the con-gregation was singing a song also; it drowned him out. I was praying that he'd stop singing by the time we did. He did. What a relief! It would have been extremely em-barrassing.

Recently, Grandpa has been in the hospital two times. The first time he had pneumonia. This shocked his whole system and stopped his intestines from working, which gave him a bad pain in his stomach.

The second time Grandpa was ill, I came home from school one day and I knew at once that something was wrong with him because he had his shirt off, and he just looked different. When I asked him what was wrong, he held his hand to his lower stomach and told me how much it hurt. He sat there and moaned; he was in more pain than I have seen anyone else in.

I talked to my mom about it, and she said that Grandpa had been complaining for an hour. I thought we should take him to the hospital right away. My mom thought differently. She thought that he was exaggerating his pain and that just because his stomach hurt a little we shouldn't rush him off to the doctor. She said that when I'm sick we don't jump to the doctor's office.

She didn't seem to care! She just washed her hair, acting like nothing was wrong. This really annoyed me! I was infuriated. Grandpa exaggerates all his emotions — but this doesn't mean he doesn't have them!

She thought he was having gallbladder problems or a gallstone. She did finally call my aunt Betty (a nurse) and then the doctor. He prescribed some medication, assuming the problem was gallbladder, or whatever.

Meanwhile Grandpa went through periods of great (moaning) pain. Then he was asking for a doctor. He wanted one right away, and we didn't seem to be trying to get him one. So he fought to get outside. He was going to "run away" and ask someone on the street to take him to the hospital.

Then he lay down for a while, from five o'clock till eight. While he lay there, he said very negative things like "What's the sense to live for? I'd rather die," "Give me some poison so I'll die; it's better than suffering," and "Kill me! I'd rather be dead."

Then for a while he wanted to lash out at us for his pain and said things like "You got what you wanted—I'm sick," and "You people just want to make me sick."

He said lots of things like that, blaming his sickness on us, as though we wanted it. After a while, he calmed down. I kissed him goodnight.

The next day Grandpa was worse. My dad was out of town, so my mom and Mike took him to the hospital at about seven o'clock in the evening. At ten o'clock my mom called and said that they had taken Grandpa into emergency to do tests, and she and Mike hadn't see him since.

That was the saddest thing! Poor Grandpa must have been so confused, because he didn't know anyone, and no one knew how to handle him.

I postponed writing about Grandpa's sickness because I refused to believe in and accept his sickness. I hoped that nothing would come of it. I wanted him to be like he was before!

I can't imagine life without Grandpa. What an empty home this will be.

Emily Dickinson wrote a poem that says, "Had I not seen the sun/ I could have borne the shade. . . . "*

Since Grandpa has come here, I will really miss him when he goes. If Grandpa dies, it will be a loss for me, but it will probably be a gain for him; anyway, what happens, happens.

Today is Sunday. Just a while ago, I was doing homework, and my dad was watching Grandpa. Grandpa was saying that he had to go home, that this wasn't where he lived. My dad was explaining over and over that, yes, Grandpa does live here. This way of talking to and handling Grandpa, I've realized long ago, does not work. Grandpa was feeling like he doesn't belong here. Getting angry and impatient with his insistence on going home only make things worse. If, instead of that, I talk, laugh, and pay attention to him, he forgets all about going home.

So I took some time out of homework to cheer Grandpa up. I talked to him a while. He pointed out that it was windy outside. The trees were waving slightly.

Then he said, "Hey, I haven't been out yet. I'm gonna look outside."

"Yeah, let's go for a walk."

---

*Thomas H. Johnson, ed., *Complete Poems of Emily Dickinson* (Boston: Little, Brown, 1960), poem no. 1233.

"No, no." Back to despondent mood. He usually won't go for a walk. He thinks he's too weak.

"Come on; it's real nice out, like a spring day!" I said to him. He got up and went to the door. I grabbed his cap.

"No, I don't need that."

"Come on."

He stopped and buttoned up the top button on his shirt. I put up the hood on my sweatshirt jacket.

"No, it's not that cold!"

"Mm hm." It was January.

We started out. He took a few great gasps of air, enjoying it. "Fresh air!"

It was so funny, I imitated him. A short distance away was a small puddle from the melting snow. The rest of the driveway was dry. "Let's take a walk to the puddle!"

"Mupple?"

"No, the water. Let's take a few steps." (I pointed.) It was windy.

"Cold!"

"Yeah. I'll get our coats."

"Naw! Don't do that. I won't be out long."

"If I get them, we can stay out longer!"

"No."

"Wait one second." I dashed to the house, grabbed our coats, and came back.

"Oh! My!"

We put them on. My dad and Cindy came out to walk to the store. My dad threw a snowball at us. It must have scared Grandpa, because he can't move fast and run away or fight back. I grabbed a handful of snow and threw back at them. We had a great fight, Dad and Cindy against me! Boy, my aim is bad!

It ended when Grandpa called out, "For shame! Two men against one!"

I ran back over to him, and Dad and Cindy went to

the store. He was a little angry at them, even after my assurance that it was all in fun.

"Let's go inside," he told me.

It was a lot of fun talking to Grandpa outside and looking at the trees, snow, cars, and people. I really appreciate him a lot more when we do things like that together.

I've noticed that many persons, but especially the elderly, have characteristics that are special to them alone, whether it's the twist of an eyebrow or a special handshake. My Grandpa has lots of these things. He has a fantastic wave that he uses as a greeting or a goodbye. It's sort of like an army salute, but he makes a certain jerk of his hand when he does it. I love it. I try to copy it, but it looks rather out of place on me.

He also has his caps. They are made of a tweed cloth, round, with a little visor for the front. Grandpa has a precise way of putting his cap on. If I put it on for him, he always removes it and puts it on for himself. He sets it on the top of his head, then firmly tugs it forward and down. He really looks distinguished in it.

Grandpa's corncob pipe is very characteristic of him. He has a certain way of stuffing tobacco in it, and of lighting it. Then he pokes the tobacco down with his finger and the flame goes out, so he has to light it again and again. He says he doesn't smoke much, but he sure enjoys his pipe. He calls it his friend. He even has a permanent blister or bump on his tongue where his pipe touches it.

One day, I asked Grandpa, "Will you do me a favor?"

"Sure."

"Sign your name on this page. Right there."

"No, I won't do that!"

"Why not? Come on!" I wrote his name so he could see how.

"No, I did that before, and they got thirty? thirty-eight? thirty-eight dollars from me. I'm not going to do that! I'm sorry, I don't sign my name for no one."

"I just want it for your fancy signature."

"No, they cheat me."

"No!"

"Yes, they do; they take my property."

So I guess I don't have his signature for my book! I wanted it because it is so beautiful. He makes elaborate capital letters that he learned in Czechoslovakia. Now he is forgetting so many things, I am afraid he will forget his special way of signing his name.

Since Grandpa wouldn't sign his name, I asked him if I could draw his picture. He said, "Sure." I put a lamp on the table so that it made his shadow on the wall. I drew his silhouette on a large piece of paper. Later my mom scaled it down for me.

It seems strange, but before Grandpa came to live with us, I hadn't known him at all. In these past two years, so many things have happened that now I just think he's the greatest!

The approach of the second spring and summer since Grandpa's arrival found Milt and me with heavy hearts. We failed to share much of Terese's positive attitude toward Grandpa. I was with him so much that I could feel my patience ebbing each day from morning on, so that by evening I was exhausted. Milt's problem was exaggerated by the father-son relationship. His father was no longer a father at all; he had become a retarded, disobedient child. The arguments between them caused me consternation. What could we do to relieve this strain?

It was natural to begin thinking of summertime vacations—a time of escape, if only temporary. One of the community involvements that Milt and I shared at that time was a Young Life adult committee. This was a group of individuals who supported the Young Life Christian ministry to high-school youth. Our interest had begun back when our daughter Pat was in high school. She had attended a Young Life camp in Colorado for a week one summer, and it had contributed to a significant change in her life. Since our own church had no program for these young people, we saw Young Life as a viable organization worthy of support. Therefore when we were later asked to help the group as members of an Elmhurst committee for fund raising, we agreed.

It came about that some people we met on the committee told us about a fabulous vacation they had just enjoyed. It was a double vacation: they first went backpacking and primitive camping in the Colorado mountains, then spent a week of fun and leisure at Trail West Lodge, a lodge operated by Young Life near Buena Vista, Colorado. To Milt, who had had a hankering for backpacking for years, this sounded like the first level of heaven itself. The more we thought about it, the more attractive it sounded.

Milt began collecting information on primitive camping and survival skills. Terese and Cindy were excited about the possibility of going horseback riding in Colorado.

I became frantic to find a nursing home that would promise space in advance to accommodate Grandpa for two weeks or a month during July. Two weeks was all the time we needed, but I was told that, because of all the paperwork involved, the nursing homes would accept patients for a minimum of one month—if they had room. The Pinewood Nursing Home, where he had stayed before, was now full and could not guarantee that they would have space later in the year. Bed space for a man was more at a premium than bed space for a woman because the rooms were two-bed rooms, and most patients were women. After nearly exhausting the Yellow Pages, I finally located a "home" where space was available. It was located on an estate on beautifully wooded grounds. Milt and I visited there together, with Grandpa, explaining the type of care he would need, as we had done the previous summer at the other nursing home.

Confident that the arrangements were secure, I sent a deposit and made reservations for four of us for one week at Trail West Lodge. We would spend the first week at the lodge and a second week primitive camping, getting a taste of backpacking on short day-trips. This was similar to what our friends had done, but in reverse order.

Just two weeks before our scheduled departure, Cindy became very ill with a sore throat and fever. When she failed to get better, I took her to the doctor, who requested routine blood tests for "mono" and "strep." The phone call came the next day: Cindy had mononucleosis. This was a crushing blow, not only because Cindy was very ill, but because our vacation plans seemed to be going out the window.

The doctor explained to me that there is really no treatment for mono. The body heals itself with rest and fluids. I asked about the possibility of continuing with our vacation plans, and he said, "She might be able to go, but not to do anything strenuous."

We resolved to try. At this point, Cindy's throat was so swollen that she could scarcely swallow at all. She couldn't even breathe lying down, but had to be propped up on pillows in a sitting position.

I found a borrowed copy of Adele Davis's controversial book *Let's Get Well* on my bookshelf, and read what it had to say about mononucleosis.* It seemed that some cases showed marked improvement with high dosages of vitamin C at frequent intervals.

Cindy could not swallow any kind of pill, so I dissolved large quantities of chewable vitamin C tablets in orange juice and gave it to her every fifteen minutes by way of a straw. I also tried blackstrap molasses, but after the first sip Cindy would have none of that. Incredibly, two or three days later Cindy was much improved. It began to look as though we still might be able to go on our trip.

As Cindy continued to improve, and the doctor checked her over at the end of the week, we really resumed hoping. But we had to revise our plans.

First, we phoned Trail West to ask if our reservations could be changed to one week later. They could. This would give Cindy another week of recuperation.

Next we decided that Milt, Terese, and perhaps Mart would drive to Colorado for the primitive camping part of the trip, which was now rescheduled for week number one. Cindy and I would take a plane to Colorado Springs after the first week, and Mart would fly home. Then the four of us—Milt, Terese, Cindy, and I—would drive to Buena Vista for our week at the lodge. All of

*Adele Davis, *Let's Get Well* (New York: Harcourt, Brace and World, 1965).

this was unusually extravagant for our family, but taking care of Grandpa was so difficult that it made us feel we deserved a special vacation.

Before dawn on Sunday morning, the three campers left in our small Honda Civic with car carrier on top. Mart, who was working at the news agency as a driver that summer, had decided to go at the last minute without getting permission from his boss, who couldn't be located on such short notice. Milt and Mart took turns driving and travelled nonstop to Colorado. Once there, the campers followed an old logging road into a primitive area and hiked beyond where the car could go, revelling in the peace and solitude and in the untouched natural beauty of mountains, blue sky, and silvery clear streams.

Back at home, I continued to nourish Cindy with vitamin C tablets, fresh vegetables, chicken soup, and all the other good stuff I had ever heard about. One of the main ingredients of the healing treatments from the beginning had been prayer for her complete recovery. Now my prayers were filled with gratitude that the Lord was not only healing her, but that it was happening so fast, and that we could still have our long-anticipated vacation.

In the middle of the week, we received a call from Milt, inquiring how Cindy was doing, and I replied that our plans were still "go." Milt was ecstatic about the trip he and Terese and Mart were enjoying. We solidified our plans to meet at the airport in Colorado Springs at two o'clock on Saturday afternoon.

On Friday morning I packed Grandpa's clothes, each item carefully labeled with his name. On Friday afternoon Cindy, Grandpa, and I drove the several miles to the nursing home where Grandpa was to stay. We checked him into a nice room which he would share with another gentleman, who was not in the room but in the lounge, where the television was on. Several people, seemingly oblivious to it, were sitting silently around the room.

I assured Grandpa that we would be back for him in a few days, but naturally, when we were leaving, he wanted to leave with us. The woman who checked him in took him by the hand and led him back inside.

I had a sinking feeling in my stomach, yet I felt free. We stopped for ice cream on the way home. Cindy felt well again. Everything would be fine.

The next morning, before leaving for the airport, I called the nursing home to inquire about Grandpa. "He had a bad night," the attendant said, "but he's okay now." It seems he hadn't wanted to go to bed and had made somewhat of a fuss, keeping others awake. This was not surprising, since he often behaved that way at home also.

Later that morning, Mike, whose summer job left his weekends free, drove us to the airport. It was Cindy's first flight, and she was excited. The day was perfect: sunny and warm with a pleasant, cooling breeze.

We arrived at the small airport and scanned the area in vain. After we had waited for half an hour, our disreputable, scuzzy-looking relatives drove up and disembarked. Milt apologized for being late. The drive on mountain roads had taken much longer than they had expected. He had not had time to shave, and the only clean shirt Mart had to wear was one that had a large rip in the shoulder seam. Oh well, it was still good to be together again.

Terese was beaming with the experience of being so close to nature and so far from any sort of reminder of the "outside world." She loved it.

We went to the airport restaurant for a quick lunch before saying good-bye to Mart and putting him on a plane to return home. He was hoping he would still have his job. He had, however, truly enjoyed the trip. This was to be his first air flight, too: an adventure quite different from primitive camping.

After Mart's plane left, we continued on to Trail West Lodge. This lodge is owned by the Young Life ministry and operated as a place for their staff and volunteer personnel to enjoy at low cost while attending conferences or simply vacationing. The housekeeping and food preparation are done mainly by volunteer crews from Young Life youth groups throughout the United States.

To us, everything seemed nearly perfect. The accommodations were clean and attractive, the scenery incredibly beautiful, the food fantastic, and the people warm and friendly. Terese and Cindy discovered the game room right away and were soon teaching Milt and me to play pool. There was table tennis when the pool table was busy. The outdoor swimming pool was beautiful; the weather, a little too cool for swimming, was perfect for horse-back riding. The horses and the terrain were rustic and exciting— much different from the stables back home. Each evening, folks would get together to sing songs by the fireplace and eat delicious homemade ice cream.

One day there was an afternoon jaunt on "Ruby Mountain," where we hunted—and found—some small rubies embedded in the rocks. There was a whirlwind jeep caravan up to the top of a mountain for an early-morning breakfast at a small chalet; and a chuck-wagon barbecue in a beautiful aspen grove with a hilar-ious program provided by the staff.

The only part of the fun that was too strenuous for Cindy was the hike up the mountain to the site of an old gold mine. I didn't make it all the way up, myself.

We were enjoying ourselves so thoroughly that we scarcely gave a thought to those at home. However, by midweek I was feeling that we should call and find out how things were.

Mike answered the phone. At first he was vague and hesitant; then the story came out. "We didn't want you to know," he said. Grandpa was back home. The nursing home had phoned on Saturday, after I had left, and since no one was at home, they had then called our married daughter, Pat, to say that Frank was unmanageable and that the family should pick him up immedi-ately. Among other things, he had broken the glasses and sprained the wrist of one of the attendants.

This caused some degree of confusion, and ultimately a con-ference of the four older children was called, to determine what they should do. They decided first of all not to interrupt our trip. It was arranged that son-in-law John would pick Grandpa up on Sunday morning and take him to our house; Mart, who was working the morning shift from two to seven at the news agency (he had been reinstated after a stiff reprimand), would be with Grandpa during the day; Mike, who worked from eight to five daily, would be with him at night. Marian and Pat would come some evenings and on the weekend until we returned. They had an elaborate schedule worked out and posted on the refrigerator.

What myriad feelings assailed me at this news: pride and gratitude that our kids had taken charge and worked things out for us; anger that the nursing home should be so inept; amazement at the resourcefulness of Mike and Mart and their willingness to take on so much of the burden; and most of all, a surge of praise and gratitude to the Lord for his wondrous gifts.

We continued to bask in the joys of Trail West up to the moment of departure and even beyond. As we drove the 1000-plus miles home, Milt and I alternating in the driver's seat, we continued to sing the Young Life songs we had learned together at the evening sing-alongs; and so the spirit of the week remained with us all the way home. It was a beautiful ending to the summer.

Senility. Hardening of the arteries. This was the doctor's diagnosis of Grandpa's problems. But these terms did not ring true to me. I remember consulting the dictionary in frustration. Senility, according to Webster's, means old age. I knew that Grandpa was not simply old. There was something wrong with his brain that made him forget so much and act so strangely.

That fall, when Grandpa had been living with us for about a year and a half, a friend of mine said to me, "Did you read that article in the [local paper] about Alzheimer's disease?"

"No. What is that?" I had never heard the name before.

"I think it sounds like what your father-in-law has. Read the article."

I found the article, and I was totally amazed. The symptoms described were Grandpa's to a T. I was sure his problems were due to Alzheimer's disease.

Just a week later, the *Chicago Tribune* published a series of articles on Alzheimer's disease. I made sure to get every part of the series. At the end of each article was a note about an organization in the Chicago area called Alzheimer's Disease and Related Disorders Association—ADRDA. An address was listed to which one could write for more information. I sent in my name immediately, and within a short time I had received brochures, a newsletter, announcements of local speakers and events, and the name of a support group leader in my area.

Sometimes I wonder why this mattered so much to me. Knowing that Grandpa had a brain disease didn't change anything, but it did convince me that he couldn't help being the way he was. It explained why he was so out of touch with his surroundings, while many old people continued to be rational and alert into their nineties and beyond. Most importantly, it put me in touch with others who understood completely the difficulties of caring for Grandpa, because they were going through the same things with a loved one of their own.

I was excited to read about this new discovery—that Alzheimer's disease was now believed to be responsible for the irrational behavior known as senile dementia. I told Milt and the rest of the family about it and showed them the articles and information I'd received. They all agreed that the descriptions certainly sounded like Grandpa. All but Mike. He didn't believe there was anything wrong with Grandpa at all. He thought it was our fault that Grandpa was so cranky and irritable. He thought we should all pay more (much more) attention to Grandpa and then he'd be fine. Mike and I got into big arguments about this. I couldn't convince him. I guess at times Mike saw that his thinking was unrealistic, but it was the way he felt. He was simply unable to accept the sentence of Alzheimer's disease for his grandfather. Until much later.

Alzheimer's disease was discovered by a German neuropathologist, Alois Alzheimer, in 1906. He examined the brain cells of deceased persons who at the age of fifty or earlier had experienced severe memory loss, dementia, and eventual complete loss of human faculties. He found that the brains of these people contained masses of what he called "plaques and tangles," which had totally destroyed the normal cells in certain parts of the brain. Depending on the severity of the disease at the time of death, lesser or greater portions of the brain were obliterated by this strange mass.

The term "Alzheimer's disease" was first used to diagnose the symptoms of severe memory loss and dementia in people of middle age or younger. It was, however, not used at first to diagnose the same symptoms in people who were in their late sixties and older. Many doctors and others believed that these symptoms were an almost inevitable result of the aging process.

The terms "senility" and "senile dementia" were used to diagnose the symptoms. "Hardening of the arteries in the brain" and "organic brain syndrome" were designated as causes. Scientific developments in the late 1970s led to greater use of diagnostic testing of the brain. As a result, older people with severe memory loss and dementia were being given thorough batteries of tests that identified the nonfunctioning areas of the brain. These tests could rule out all known diseases but often failed to identify the cause of the symptoms.

Meanwhile, pathological research had revealed that the brain cells of many aged persons who had symptoms of senile dementia were similar to the cells of younger people who had died with Alzheimer's disease. Thus diagnostic testing became important in identifying Alzheimer's by a process of elimination. If the person had no other identifiable disease (many diseases have similar symptoms), then he or she could be said to have Alzheimer's disease, although there was no infallible way to confirm the diagnosis until after death, when a brain autopsy could be performed.

Even though I didn't take Grandpa for these diagnostic tests, when I read the symptoms of the disease—loss of memory, especially about recent events; disorientation in what were once familiar surroundings; extreme irritability; and poor judgment in caring for oneself—I recognized them in Grandpa. As we watched Grandpa and listened to him speak, we could see that he was forgetting many words, especially nouns, although he'd get around the problem somehow, by motions or by using descriptive words. He had forgotten how to tell time. He still looked at the clock, but now he couldn't tell one hand from the other. It might be two-thirty and he'd say, "Oh, my! Six o'clock!" Of course, his insistence on going home was totally irrational. In my opinion, this couldn't be an inevitable occurrence of aging. (The diagnosis of Alzheimer's disease was eventually confirmed by a neurologist.)

Very soon after receiving the brochures from the ADRDA, I attended a support-group meeting in a nearby city. The group was fairly new, led by a woman whose mother had recently been diagnosed as having Alzheimer's disease. The mother was unable to live alone and was now living with her daughter and son-in-law and their two children. The support group consisted of ten or twelve others who were in similar situations or had someone in a nursing home. Meetings were held in a church at six-week intervals, and there was no fee.

At first, after learning about the ADRDA, I went to the support-group meetings alone or with one of my friends from RE:AL who was interested. When I came home, I would tell Milt about it, but he showed no interest in attending these meetings himself. He stayed home with Grandpa. The primary function of the meetings was to provide each participant with the opportunity to tell the group what was happening with his or her "patient": any changes that had taken place, any especially exasperating things that had happened, any questions that had arisen, or any problems that needed to be solved. As each person told his or her story, others chimed in with their experiences, questions, and suggestions. Everyone could feel the empathy and understanding of the group members. The group leader was careful to allow each person time to speak. Then, over coffee, people sought out those whose experience most closely related to their own, for more discussion. Occasionally a speaker was invited to talk about some particular area such as legal assistance, Medicare, or social security. People shared sources of information such as where to ask for home care, which nursing homes would accept Alzheimer patients, how to get dental care, and which doctors were knowledgeable about Alzheimer's disease. For many people, the support group was the only social activity they had, since they could seldom leave their patient.

The Alzheimer's Disease and Related Disorders Association (ADRDA) was organized in 1979.* It emphasized support groups from the very beginning, and these were the basis for its growth. The national association soon led to regional associations, which provided members with periodic newsletters, information about

*The Alzheimer's Disease and Related Disorders Association, Inc., 70 East Lake Street, Chicago, Illinois 60601.

family support groups, and notification about public meetings with speakers and panel discussions, all done by volunteers. Volunteer support has been very helpful in publicizing the name of the disease and the need for research. For example, the late Rita Hayworth, the Hollywood starlet of the '40s and 50s, suffered from Alzheimer's disease at the end of her life, and her daughter has been a strong advocate of the ADRDA.

The media have continued to make the public aware of this disease and of the need for research into its cause and treatment. The basic reason, though, for the spread of concern about Alzheimer's disease is that it affects so many people either directly — through a close relative or friend — or indirectly. I believe it is the prevalence and severity of the problem that accounts for the urgency of the search for solutions. While the search goes on, however, families like ours continue to grapple with the destruction caused by the disease.

That fall, as I was learning about Alzheimer's disease and ADRDA, Terese turned sixteen and got her driver's license and her first job, at McDonald's. Cindy joined the seventh-grade cross country team and became the number one girl runner. In midyear Mart transferred from Northern Illinois University to the University of Wisconsin, Green Bay, more than two hundred miles from home, where he planned to major in environmental studies. Mike was looking forward to graduation from Northern Illinois University in May with a degree in biology, but he was not quite sure what to do with it. He applied to do some volunteer work in deprived areas of the United States and waited to see what would come of the application.

Years that had previously sped by seemed now to go much more slowly. The days were long and difficult. Milt and I continued our involvements in evening activities whenever we could, especially with our church. I was always on the lookout for possible sitters, but I could usually count on tucking Grandpa into bed at seven o'clock. Terese or Cindy would be home with him, so Milt and I felt free to leave. Occasionally we would come home to find him up and restless, and Terese or Cindy complaining,

"Grandpa's a pain! I couldn't get my homework done." Then I felt guilty. Moreover, one time Grandpa became very angry with Cindy for some reason and forced her to go outside. She sat on the stone railing on the carport, waiting. Meanwhile Terese, hearing the hubbub, came downstairs and found Grandpa pressing the back of a chair under the doorknob. After a few minutes his anger cooled, and Cindy came back inside. I felt a lot of guilt when I found out that this had happened, but there was never any threat of physical harm, so I did nothing about it. Both Terese and Cindy knew how to handle Grandpa: to entertain and cajole him, not to try to coerce him in any way. If he became hostile, they knew enough to stay away from him. It didn't happen often, though, and I couldn't see the need to hire a sitter when Grandpa was asleep and the girls were home. More and more often it was just Cindy who was at home. Terese's part-time job and other activities kept her busy. I didn't realize the difficult position Cindy was in when I'd ask, "Is it okay if I go to such-and-such tonight, Cindy? You'll be home, won't you, if Grandpa gets up?"

Grandpa continued to be lonely in our midst, bewildered, not sure who we were or where he would sleep at night. He sometimes laughed and made jokes, but at other times he was irritable and easily angered. Basically, he had a grateful heart and often thanked us sincerely for whatever we did for him.

Grandpa sat in the kitchen. He had finished his snack and looked up at the clock. "Six o'clock! My, I didn't know it was so late."

"It's not six o'clock, Grandpa, it's only two-thirty. See?" I pointed to the hour hand.

"Oh, yes." He was quiet for a moment, looking out the window. "Well, I hafta go now. It's six o'clock." He got up slowly.

"I just told you, Grandpa. It's only two-thirty. It's not six o'clock yet." He stood at the window watching some sparrows flitting about in the shrubs.

"They won't come to me. They don't like me."

I looked up from the letter I was writing to see what he meant. "Grandpa, they don't even know you're there. They're just birds looking for food."

"Well, it's late. I hafta go home."

"This is your home. You don't have to go anywhere, Grandpa. You live here."

"No, this is not my home. My wife is there, waiting for me. I have to go."

I didn't like the way this conversation was going. How could I convince him? "What don't you like about this place, Grandpa?"

"I don't know. I have to go home."

"You are home already. Why don't you just smoke your pipe?"

"My pipe? Smoke? I don't know where it is."

"I'll get it for you. Come on." He followed me to his room, lit his pipe, and sat in the foyer smoking it, since it was too cold to go outside.

"I don't smoke much," he said. "I used to smoke cigarettes, but they cost too much money. I like my pipe. That's my good friend." He stroked it gently, then put it back in his mouth. He seemed content.

Early one Saturday morning, when I had given up trying to sleep late and instead sat in the kitchen with Grandpa, encouraging him to tell me about his memories, Milt, also awake, was upstairs listening. As I was prompting Grandpa to tell me his familiar stories, sometimes he would say, "I don't know; I can't remember" about things he had often told us before. Milt realized that Grandpa was beginning to lose some of these memories of his early years—his childhood in Czechoslovakia, crossing the Atlantic Ocean as a boy of twelve, growing up in America. Milt had the idea of compiling these simple narratives in a loose-leaf notebook in the form of Grandpa's autobiography, so that as Grandpa read them over and over, his memory of these events would be refreshed. He wrote the words with felt-tip pen in large, easy-to-read letters that Grandpa could read even without his glasses. The book began with the date of Frank's birth; it included the names of his parents, brother, and sisters, and the town where he lived in Czechoslovakia. It recounted the little stories he had told us so many times about his boyhood, the journey across the ocean, his schooling, his job, his marriage, the birth of his son, and the homes they lived in. It also included his son's (Milt's) marriage, the birth of his grandchildren, and the death of his wife; it told how he lived alone for many years and then came to live with his son and our family. This was an attempt, on Milt's part, to both preserve Grandpa's history and to provide a stimulant for his memory as it continued to wane.

This book became a constant companion. Grandpa would be content to sit and read—even though sometimes he was only mouthing the words out loud—either by himself or with someone to sit and encourage him.

Often the words he read would trigger the memory, and he would look up and talk from his recollections, using the same words each time.

We left the book on the family-room table in the evening so Grandpa would find it in the morning and entertain himself for a while after he had his apple or early-morning snack. When we had to take him shopping, to a doctor's appointment, or anywhere which required an extended drive, we would take his book along and encourage him to read it. He would sit alone and read out loud to himself. He enjoyed it most, however, if we asked him to read to us. He didn't seem to know or care that we had heard it all hundreds of times before.

One evening Terese had brought some balloons home from McDonald's, and she and Cindy were tossing them around. Grandpa began tapping them back when they came his way. Another valuable pastime had been discovered. Everyone in the family learned to get a balloon volley going whenever Grandpa's evening restlessness would start, or when he indicated that he was tired or bored. We kept a supply of balloons handy—mostly free advertising from certain stores—and Terese found that the tiny rubber bands left over from when she had braces on her teeth were perfect for tying the balloons so that they could be reused. This game gave Grandpa excellent exercise for his arms and also stimulated hand/eye coordination.

Occasionally in the evening Cindy, Grandpa, and I played a card game of rummy together. It was a little frustrating when Grandpa failed to follow the rules! Cindy, who is a very competitive card player, found it hard to give up winning so that Grandpa could be entertained.

Until this time, Grandpa had used the bathroom in privacy.

However, once in a while I discovered that strange things were going on in there. One day I found that he had taken the bar of soap and tried to eat it. Another time, someone had left some liquid laundry soap on the sink; Grandpa opened it and tasted it—then complained loudly that someone had given it to him to poison him. We had to keep all soap in the cupboard where he would not notice it. The towel was always missing. Grandpa would stuff it into his pocket (perhaps torn in half) or hide it elsewhere. Finally I couldn't leave a towel in his bathroom any longer. I also removed the pictures from the wall because he would take them. Most annoying, the waste basket was found to have urine in it several times, so it had to be removed. When I failed to watch Grandpa closely enough, he sometimes used the corner of his bedroom or the closet floor for a urinal. He seldom, if ever, flushed the toilet, but sometimes he would "wash his hands" in the toilet water, so I had to monitor him constantly. Eventually, Milt helped us to prevent some of these aberrations by installing a little bell above the bathroom door. This was a simple means to make sure Grandpa's visits were supervised. I would open the closed door just enough to make sure he was doing the proper things, but letting him think he had privacy.

Grandpa's sleep habits changed gradually. Once he got to sleep at night, he still slept until morning, but from early dusk on he became increasingly restless. "I've got to be getting home," he'd say, looking at the clock in the kitchen. He'd prowl around the house, becoming visibly and audibly more agitated, and we'd take turns trying various methods to distract him. Normally he would be tired and ready to go to bed by seven o'clock, but sometimes he decided he didn't want to go to bed, which was most aggravating.

I depended upon routine for stability. Even a slight change, like the turning of clocks an hour ahead in the spring, was enough to disrupt our evening ritual for what seemed like weeks at a time. Dinner was from five to six o'clock, allowing an hour for relaxation and kitchen cleanup before Grandpa's bedtime at seven. After the time change, Grandpa was noticeably unready to settle down at seven o'clock, which was really six. It was still broad daylight at that time.

When we moved the clocks back in the fall, the problem was just the reverse. Grandpa could not wait for dinner and kept demanding snacks, until by dinner time he was no longer hungry and couldn't stay awake. If he went to bed at five-thirty or fell asleep in a chair, after a half-hour's nap he'd be up for hours, pestering and demanding attention one way or another.

One spring day had been a difficult one for me, so after dinner I was happy to hear Milt say, "I'll put Grandpa to bed, Rosalie." (As when our children were small, I was usually the one who took care of the bedtime ritual.) It was almost seven o'clock.

"Come with me, Dad," Milt said, and took Grandpa's hand to help him up from his chair.

"Who, me? What for?"

"It's time to get ready for bed now."

"Yeah? I'm not sleepy."

"Come on, Dad." Milt's voice was louder, more intense. "Let's go!" He reached one arm around Grandpa's back and forced him to his feet. Then he pulled him by the hand.

"No! I don't want to!"

Mike came into the kitchen and witnessed the scuffle. "You shouldn't treat Grandpa that way. Why don't you wait awhile? Maybe he'll change his mind."

"No, I don't believe in waiting for him. Come on, Dad. Now!"

Mike walked away with a sigh.

Grandpa shuffled along reluctantly. When they got to the bedroom, Milt's commands continued.

"Take off your shirt, Dad."

"No. I won't!"

"Yes, you will." Milt began unbuttoning the shirt and finally got it off. Milt's authoritative manner was one he had learned from his father years ago; it had persisted, though considerably mellowed, through parenting six children. Now he and his father were subjects of a role reversal, and the old pattern of "I'm the boss" returned in full force, with Milt insisting on winning the power struggle.

"Now take your pants off, please." Milt unfastened the belt. Grandpa opened the fly and let his pants fall.

"Sit down." The words were accompanied with strong pressure on Grandpa's shoulders.

Grandpa sat on the bed. Milt slipped the shoes and pants off and handed the pajamas bottoms to Grandpa. Slowly he arranged the opening in front of him, lifted one foot, then the other, Milt standing by impatiently.

"Okay, put this on now." Milt held the pajama top so Grandpa could put it on while seated.

"Good. Now stand up." They finished buttoning everything. "Now let's go to the bathroom." Grandpa complied, and Milt sat reading the newspaper while Grandpa took his time in the bathroom. When he came out, Milt ushered him back to the bedroom and tucked him into bed.

"Goodnight, Dad. God bless you."

"Goodnight," came the sullen reply.

A few minutes later, we could hear Grandpa talking to himself. Soon he was in the hall. Milt went to meet him and guided him back to the bathroom, again reading while he waited. I had gone down to the rec room in the basement to watch a television program.

Finally, Grandpa came out and was again ushered back to bed. Milt came down to watch TV with me.

Soon Grandpa was up again, walking around and talking to himself. "Where are they? Nobody," we could hear him say. When the next commercial came on, Milt went back to go through the scenario again. Then I took a turn. Our assumption was that perhaps Grandpa's inability to sleep was connected with a need to use the bathroom. Whether this was accurate or not, there was some comfort in following the routine. Another hour went by with Grandpa alternately in bed and bathroom. Finally he was quiet, but Milt and I both felt that we had been robbed of a pleasant evening.

Like many traditional homemakers, I have lived most of my adult life as a person who serves others—husband and children— giving first priority to their needs and demands. Consequently, feelings of resentment have often been my particular demon.

These feelings were buried so deeply that they seldom surfaced, but I knew their signs: the heaviness, the lack of joy, the sudden sharp words that came with slight provocation. Through various studies and growth experiences over the past several years, I had gained a good deal of insight and self-awareness and had been freed of much of that resentment. Now I was determined not to let it recur as I took care of Grandpa. After all, responding to the necessity was something that I chose to do. Fortunately, I had the support of Milt and my family, but at times it wasn't enough.

The greatest difficulty with resentment came when Milt continued his enjoyment of outdoor activities and I automatically agreed to "stay home with Grandpa," his father. On the one hand, I did want him to take the children skiing, for example, to utilize two or three days during the Christmas holiday; but, on the other hand, I felt that heaviness of spirit, a tightening in my stomach, that told me I was not really free of that old demon.

Toward the end of the second year Grandpa lived with us, Milt and Terese made plans to go canoeing during the Easter holiday (consulting me first, of course). It was a trip that I really encouraged, since I knew it would be a beautiful father-daughter experience, yet I wished that there were somewhere that I wanted to go, too. But there wasn't. Home was where I wanted to be. So why the bitter feeling?

I had begun writing about Grandpa when the mood struck me. It felt good to put down on paper what was happening in my life. An example:

> After being busy elsewhere in the house, I enter the room where Grandpa is. "You know," he begins a familiar theme, "there were times—I don't know how far back it was—there were times when I was all alone. Two, three days, all alone. I was so lonely I could cry. Were you ever alone?"
>
> "Yes, Grandpa, but not as much as you. You lived alone for nine years."
>
> "I don't know how far back it was, I was here all alone."
>
> "That was before you came here, Grandpa. Yes, you

were alone for a long time. How does it feel to be alone?"

"Bad. I feel bad. I got nobody. Nothing. I'm all alone."

"I'm sorry, Grandpa. You can stay here with me. Then we'll be together, okay?"

"You're a good girl. Thank you." He reached for my hand and kissed it tenderly.

6 · The Third Year

As we began the third year of Grandpa's care, it seemed that our family had settled into a routine of treating Grandpa as an accepted member of the family. We were familiar with his moods and had learned to respond to his needs. For me, he was the main focus of my life. There was nothing I could do or think without considering him—making sure that he was dressed and fed and comfortable, that he had something to do, that there was someone looking after him if I was not. I coordinated all the family activities, trying to maintain harmony, making sure Grandpa wasn't lost in the shuffle.

That year, Mike completed his studies at Northern Illinois University early in May and moved back home. Mike's application to do volunteer work for a year had led nowhere. He was not qualified to teach, and although he knew a lot about ornithology and biology and had lots of good intentions, no one needed what he had to offer. Instead he worked as a counselor at the Elmhurst YMCA day camp for a second summer, while looking into jobs involving a biology background.

Mart, attending the University of Wisconsin, Green Bay, reported that he liked Wisconsin life much better than "suburbia." He took a summer job as a counselor also, at a "Y" camp north of Green Bay. We wouldn't see him until he made a short visit in September.

Terese, still punching the time clock part-time at McDonald's, was looking forward to spending one week of her summer at a conservation camp at Western Illinois University in Macomb. Soon to be a senior in high school, she was interested in nature and, like Mike, was looking for ways to express that interest.

Cindy had found a niche for herself in cross-country and track. Her long legs and stamina gave her a chance to compete successfully and gain praise for her efforts. Her track meets were numerous during May, and I attended as often as I could, taking Grandpa with me. Usually he stayed in the car. Cindy's friend Krista was also a runner, and the two girls were close competitors who took pleasure in urging each other on.

In June, Grandpa suffered a bladder infection and spent one week in the hospital. When he returned, he walked more slowly, talked less with other people, and stayed more to himself. We were not sure whether it was a temporary setback or part of a gradual decline.

Beginning the previous fall and all through winter and early spring, Milt had been collecting books and materials on backpacking trails and equipment. He had obtained catalogs listing the very latest in one-burner stoves, lightweight tents, polypropylene pads for sleeping, pure wool fabrics for warmth and moisture resistance, and on and on. He wanted very much to go backpacking that summer.

My own thoughts about all this were fraught with anxiety. What about Grandpa? I checked with the nursing homes in our area again, but I was not surprised that they were filled and could not promise space for respite care, especially for a man. Needless to say, I did not contact the place that had failed so miserably to serve us the summer before. From a string of leads gathered from Yellow Pages listings, newspaper ads, and public facilities, I called agencies that supposedly provided in-home care. What looked good on paper proved to be unavailable or outrageously expensive. Grandpa didn't need a skilled nurse. He just needed a housekeeper-companion. But there was none. I found this very frustrating. We were a family that simply had to have at least a short getaway vacation. We had to find some way to arrange for respite care if Grandpa was to stay with us; and there seemed to be no reason not to have him remain with us.

My volunteer work at RE:AL provided the answer. One of the women who often helped with the newsletter mailings became familiar with Grandpa as I brought him to the center with me.

Eventually, she sat with him on an afternoon or two, and he took a liking to her. She was very warm and motherly to him. Sometime in early spring I broached the idea to Mary of staying with Grandpa while we went on vacation. She considered the proposal carefully and finally agreed to take care of him mornings and afternoons for one week. That meant I had to solicit help from Mike, and also Marian and Pat, to fill in the evenings and weekend hours. They agreed. Terese and Cindy would accompany us on the trip. It seemed incredible to me that things had worked out.

Milt was overjoyed that we were going to be free to have at least a week away together. He was still more pleased when I agreed to try backpacking on a trail, which would involve carrying all necessary equipment and food, hiking several miles from one campsite to another, spending the night, continuing to the next site, and so on, in a circle which would end at the starting point. Terese reserved time out from her summer job, happy to participate in any outdoor adventure. Cindy, however, was not enthusiastic. She had only begun to learn that she could dissent from family decisions and had let her abhorrence of spiders influence her opinion of camping. But her usual habit of compliance, plus some promises of movie and pizza nights interspersed with the camping, enticed her into agreement. Milt proceeded to buy or borrow the equipment we would need and to plan the details. I was about to have my first backpacking adventure! I wasn't ecstatic about it, but it was worth a try, for the sake of a family vacation. We took a few short practice hikes to break in our new hiking boots.

The time available to us was one week during August; and because it was so short a time, Milt decided we would stay fairly close to home. He chose his favorite winter camping grounds, Kettle Moraine State Forest in Wisconsin. (For several years he had winter-camped and cross-country skied there during the Christmas–New Year break from school, usually with two or three of our children and some hardy friends.)

It proved to be a poor choice because of the heat and humidity in Wisconsin at that time of year. Swarms of mosquitoes added to the discomfort. The four of us, tenderfeet all except for Milt, trudged along with our thirty-pound packs (Milt's was probably fifty pounds or more) in alternating rain and steamy heat, all but breathing the pesky mosquitoes that fought to bite us in spite of the armor of repellent we wore. No one spoke. We just endured silently until, after three hours, Milt said, "Well, I can see this isn't going to work. Let's find a highway and I'll hitch a ride back to the car."

With that incentive we followed gladly until we came to a highway. It wasn't long before a car large enough to accommodate all four of us plus our packs stopped, and the driver generously gave us a lift back to the park headquarters and our car. We soon found an open campground where the air was clear and free of bugs, plunked ourselves down with our dried, unrefrigerated foods, and spent a relaxing week, taking short hikes without our packs, reading, singing around our evening campfires, and spending one evening in town for a pizza dinner and a movie. For Cindy and me, our introduction to backpacking became a relieved farewell.

The care of Grandpa at home had worked out well. My friend Mary had Grandpa well in hand. He helped her vacuum the floors and chop vegetables; he entertained her with his singing. She mothered him and loved him, and he was happy, with the exception of the inevitable hyper, agitated times. Mike gave generously of himself, spending each weekday evening with Grandpa, helping him to bed for the night, and being there in the morning before leaving for work.

Since we had left on a Tuesday, I had made arrangements for Marian and Pat to take their turns with Grandpa on the weekend. Pat came on Saturday morning and stayed with him all day. Mike was busy elsewhere, so she was home alone with him. She tried very hard to be nice to him—listening to his talk, fixing food for him constantly, following him around to make sure he was okay. He still wasn't satisfied, however, and in the afternoon he started insisting that he wanted to go home. I had told both girls to just bolt the doors when that happened, so Pat did. But Grandpa became very angry, yelling names at her and pounding on the door, looking very fierce. Not being used to his insults and angry words, she burst into tears and telephoned her sister Marian, sobbing, "I don't know what to do! What'll I do?"

Marian couldn't understand what there was to be upset about. "Just lock the door and stay away from him," she advised. "He'll get over it."

The next day it was Marian's turn. Again Grandpa was restless, this time getting into things. He took some mail from the desk and was stuffing it into his pockets; he picked up a glass dish from the kitchen and went to his bedroom with it, to hide it in his drawer; he began to wrap his bread and jelly snack in a piece of newspaper—he was a continuous challenge. The more Marian corrected him for taking things he shouldn't have, the angrier he got and the more trouble he seemed to find. Finally he was in the foyer trying to put the ashtray into his pocket. Marian took it away from him and pushed him out the door and closed it, locking him outside. He stood there banging on the door with his fist and shouting "Let me in, damn you, I want in!"

This time it was Marian who phoned Pat in desperation. "I've locked Grandpa outside, and he's banging on the door! What'll I do now?" They laughed together over the irony of the situation and decided that from then on, whenever they took care of Grandpa they would do it together instead of dealing with him alone. For me, it was heartwarming to see this reliance and cooperation among sisters who had at times been rivals while growing up.

On the day after we returned from our family trip, I left for Green Lake, Wisconsin, where, with a friend from RE:AL, I attended a Christian Writers' Conference. Milt still had five days of vacation left, so he was able to stay with Grandpa. The conference was such a marvelous experience for me that I looked forward to doing it again the following summer. Writing had long been an interest and a hobby of mine. Being with others of similar bent and in a beautiful setting did wonders for my soul. The conference became an annual retreat for me, a special vacation of my own, giving me nourishment for the year that followed. My unspoken wish for a place where I could go for fulfillment had come true.

I came home to a great fanfare: a six-by-four-foot sign reading Welcome Home Rosalie was tacked to the outside of the house, and some twenty little love notes from Milt were tucked here and there for me to find as I traced my way around inside. I definitely felt appreciated.

Grandpa registered no surprise at seeing me. He seemed just the same. He had a tantrum when Milt got out the ladder to take down the sign. He was sure Milt was going to rob him with that ladder going up to the window.

Grandpa was becoming weaker both physically and mentally. It was sad to hear him struggling to cut his wood, unable to decide where to make his cut. He made so many markings that it became impossible to decipher them. He kept coming to me and asking where he should cut, still frustrated after I showed him. When he finally began sawing, he tired after a few strokes and had to stop. He hid the clamp among the clothes in his dresser, hid the saw in his closet. Then he couldn't find them and accused me or someone else of stealing them. They became objects to look for rather than to use, still frustrating him. Eventually I put them away in the basement. It marked the end of a phase.

Grandpa's smoking—especially his using matches—had come into question a number of times. "Aren't you afraid he'll start a fire in that planter?" my sister Betty asked when she saw the way Grandpa lit his pipe beside it again and again. The large planter in the foyer was banked with bark chips where the plant used to be. But Grandpa's habitual cautiousness reassured me. He set the used match on the stone, rather than on the wooden table or in the ash tray. One evening when Cindy was with him, however, he lit the plastic lid of my coffee carafe instead of his pipe. Fortunately Cindy was right there and took care of it before there was serious harm to him or the kitchen. I was promptly convinced that it was time to take the matches away! From then on, whenever Grandpa wanted to smoke his pipe, he had to call one of us to light a match for him. He had forgotten the word *match* but would symbolize it by making the motion of striking one. While he smoked, it was necessary to keep running back and forth with the matches each time the pipe went out, which seemed to be whenever Grandpa packed the tobacco down with his finger. We were a family of nonsmokers, and I found it hard to tolerate this annoyance, but it did help Grandpa to pass the time.

Once a week or so, Milt lathered up Grandpa's beard and shaved him. Grandpa didn't fuss too much, but he didn't like it. Sometimes he wanted to quit when Milt was only half finished. He would, however, meekly allow Milt to continue. Haircuts were always my specialty, going back many years. "Don't be particular," he always said, "just cut it all off!" Grandpa was very patient with the haircutting. Afterward, he always expressed his gratitude for these things that we did for him. Our friends marvelled that he was such a good-natured man, and it was true, in spite of his illness.

Except for his increasingly frequent trips around the neighborhood when he was agitated and wanted to "go home," Grandpa was not very active. Much of his time was spent just sitting, talking to himself, and looking out the window. When prompted, he would still read his book, talk about his pictures or the weather, toss a balloon back and forth, peel apples or potatoes for me, or sing his melodies.

Mike now began to take more time to talk with Grandpa. When his summer job ended, Mike had been without work. He had applied for jobs in several forest preserves, but none was available. After one of Milt's teachers had mentioned that a school-bus company was in need of drivers, Mike had applied and had been hired to drive behavior-disordered children to and from a special school. He worked for about three hours in the early morning and three hours in late afternoon, with about three hours at home in between. It was a job that required a certain amount of patience and regard for young adolescents, and Mike found it to be a continuous challenge. On the whole, he liked the job. It didn't pay well, but at this time Mike was not too concerned about money.

I found it to my advantage to have Mike at home during the middle of the day. He still refused to be pinned down in advance, but if he was available when I asked him to stay with Grandpa, he was kind enough to do so. Just having another person there to break the monotony was a big help.

Mike noticed that Grandpa liked looking out of the window, so, being an avid birder, he bought some bird feeders and hung them by the windows where Grandpa usually sat—one at the dining room window and one at the family room window. It amused Grandpa for long periods to see the birds flying about and fighting with one another. Although Mike put out special combinations of seeds to attract certain species, it didn't matter to Grandpa whether the birds were sparrows, chickadees, or cardinals. Seeing their wings fluttering as they competed for a place to perch, he would call to me, "Come here! Look at that! See? They're fighting!" He wanted me to come running to see this spectacle over and over again. Sometimes he attempted to catch the birds through the glass. He resented it that they would fly away when he approached. "Well, all right," he'd say, "if they don't want to hold still, let them go. I wanted to catch them and bring them in, where it's warm."

Mike paid a lot of attention to Grandpa, and they became real pals. Each time he came home, Mike would put out his hand to Grandpa for their special handshake. He would make some joke or tease Grandpa about something so they could laugh together. It worked well. Grandpa had always loved to tease others, and he enjoyed the little jokes. "Where shall we go, Grandpa? To the moon?" or "I'll bet you're looking for your girl friend out there, aren't you?" Sometimes Grandpa came back with his own sense of humor.

Mike had evolved into the family philosopher. He had always been a sensitive youngster who cared about birds, animals, plants, and all natural things. Although Milt also saw himself as a person who cared about nature, Mike was an idealist who frequently, as he was growing up, pointed out discrepancies between our middle-class life-style and his own enlightened view of the world, and confronted his father the way only an adolescent can.

For instance, during his high-school years, there was a conflict over dandelions. When there were dandelions in the lawn, Milt thought Mike should be willing to dig them out, since he didn't approve of weed killers. But to Mike, dandelions were wildflowers that had as much right to grow as the grass! He refused on this basis or maintained he didn't have time to work on the lawn. Besides, he was highly allergic. Milt dismissed this as an excuse for laziness and considered it an affront to his authority.

At about that time, we had a problem with ants getting into

the house, and whenever Milt doused them with noxious-smelling insect spray, Mike would make dire predictions that we would poison the human race with our indiscriminate use of chemicals — however, he offered no viable alternative.

When he was a college student, Mike's favorite topic for confrontation was the failure of the United States economic and political system to provide for human and environmental needs. Milt saw Mike's views as an irresponsible assault on his patriotism as an American citizen. In a matter of moments the two could become locked in bitter debate in a futile attempt to change one another's way of thinking.

With Grandpa's entry upon this scene, Milt's dictatorial mode of operation was a ready-made opportunity for further battle. Mike, the opponent, maintained that Grandpa had a right to his own opinions, a right to dissent. He challenged Milt to back off and let Grandpa be himself, while Milt, always the authority figure, continued to use force when necessary to make this "child" behave. Trying to contend with his father's total unreasonableness was hard enough for Milt. Having to fend off a critical son at the same time was too much. Tension filled the air.

Mike's criticisms of how Grandpa was treated were not confined to Milt. He pointed out that I, too, was guilty of arguing unnecessarily with Grandpa, judging him, and criticizing him. Hearing this didn't change me at all, but it did increase my awareness and my feelings of guilt. Yet I continued to tangle with Grandpa: He was wrong. I was right. In my judgment he refused to accept the truth about himself, about us, about his situation. There was an unending debate:

"I'm going home."

"No, this is your home."

"I didn't eat nothing all day."

"You had a big breakfast one hour ago."

"There's someone coming."

"No, they're just walking by."

"I got nothing."

"You have everything you need."

"They steal."

"Nobody steals from you."

I was the expert. I knew how things were, how they should be. He had to conform.

Gradually, however, I began to ask myself, "Why? Why does Grandpa's view of reality have to conform with mine? Why do I allow myself to be drawn into arguments with him—defending myself, defending the children, scolding him for the things he does, when he so obviously needs acceptance, not criticism. Grandpa can't help this kind of behavior. What's my excuse?"

Still, it was hard to avoid the arguments, though it may sound absurd. Grandpa's mind seemed to have separate compartments. He had a number of precepts that he stated frequently, and I'm sure he believed they were true: "I don't smoke much," "I don't eat much," and "I don't swear." Making these statements seemed to satisfy a need in him; they had little or nothing to do with his behavior. For instance, he might be looking for his pipe in the afternoon or evening, and he'd say, "If I don't find it, then I won't smoke. I don't smoke much. I didn't smoke for two—three days"—when in fact he had puffed his last pipeful just half an hour before. Telling him he had smoked that day made no difference, because he didn't remember. It only made him angry. Seeing the inconsistency between his behavior and his statements aggravated me time after time. If I was already feeling irritable, it was easy to get embroiled in an argument before I could think to stop myself. On many occasions when I wanted Grandpa to go to bed so that I'd be free to leave for a meeting, I became really rough with him, pushing him down on the bed like a naughty child. At other times I let Grandpa's idiosyncrasies irritate me to the point of shouting at him or grabbing things from him unmercifully.

Our friends thought we were heroic for taking care of Milt's dad, but to me the effort to do so seemed sometimes to emphasize our worst qualities.

The ADRDA support group I had joined continued to help me deal with my guilt feelings and my frustration. So many of the people there had more difficult patients than Grandpa. One woman I often thought about was caring for her husband, who not only had Alzheimer's and could scarcely talk, but was also diabetic and a paraplegic confined to a wheelchair. He had lost his business, there was very little money, and she could not afford to put him into a nursing home without risking the loss of her home. Remembering cases like that helped to keep me from feeling too sorry for myself.

As Alzheimer's disease became a more prominent topic in the media, Milt's interest increased, and he began attending the support group meetings with me. This made them much more satisfying for me, since we both heard other peoples' stories and could react to them, and we were encouraged to talk about what we had heard.

I heard Milt report to the group that "my dad was my Rock of Gibraltar. He was never sick. He was a perfect macho type, strong, bull-headed. Now he's like a child in many ways. It's hard for me to accept that. I get so angry with him and lose my temper; and then I feel guilty."

Attending support group together meant leaving the house at about seven-fifteen in the evening, when Grandpa might or might not be in bed and asleep for the night. There were three possible sitters available—Mike, Terese, and Cindy. However, Mike had become involved in various activities and Terese had her part-time job; so more and more we relied upon Cindy, who was thirteen years old at this time. Sometimes we came home to find that Grandpa had gotten up and bothered her all evening. She complained that she wasn't able to do her homework because of him. He sat beside her at the kitchen table and criticized what she was doing: "You shouldn't put your head down so close to the paper. It's bad for your eyes." "You write too fast. You have to write slow." In addition, there was his continual stream of interruptions: "Have you got something to eat? I'm hungry." "Look how dark it is. . . . "

I knew exactly what she meant. His babble made it impossible to concentrate on anything. He bothered Cindy enough times that I began to look more seriously for occasional outside help.

There was a woman named Jane who was a member of our church community and who had stayed with Grandpa once or twice during the first year. I began calling upon her when there was an evening activity we wanted to attend. Grandpa still didn't want strangers around, but it was worth it to have her at home in case he got out of bed after we left. Most of the time he didn't, and I questioned paying her to sit and do nothing while our children were there—as if she were baby-sitting grown children! In the long run, though, I realized how much it relieved my mind to know that someone was there just for Grandpa. Ironically, there were times when she had her hands full with him—and then the children could be a great help to her.

The ADRDA support group continued to be a valuable resource for Milt and me. One piece of information we picked up from the group had to do with clothing. Until this time we had insisted that Grandpa wear pajamas to bed at night—on top of his underwear. This was now becoming a frequent source of arguments. Grandpa would refuse, I would cajole, Milt would insist; we would somehow force him into pajamas whether he wanted them or not. It was a daily hassle.

A woman in the support group said she avoided the argument over changing into night clothes with her mother by using the same clothing for daytime and nighttime. What a simple solution! But we hadn't thought of it, being caught up in the cultural routine. From that time on, Grandpa was spared the frustration of having to change his clothes before going to bed. He wore the same pants and shirt for a week at a time. He had always had a rumpled look anyway, so it didn't make any difference. What a lot of frustration it avoided for Milt and me!

People in the group sometimes talked about giving medication to their patients to prevent extreme mood swings such as those Grandpa had when he became angry and obstinate or very excited and unreasonable. It was at these times that Grandpa usually wanted to get away and would walk down the street looking for his home. It was at these times, too, that we were most frustrated because we felt Grandpa was out of our control. Milt kept asking me to take Grandpa to a doctor for medication to prevent this behavior, as others in the group apparently had done. I was reluctant, remembering that I had already confronted this problem unsuccessfully when Grandpa lived alone. However, I did make an appointment with an internist in Elmhurst. He examined Grandpa and listened to my description of the problems we were having—problems like Grandpa's outbursts of temper when he perceived something to be wrong, his overreaction to any contradiction or correction, his refusal to cooperate, his staging tantrums, threatening, and attempting to leave home, which disrupted the whole family. The doctor's response was that it seemed that sometimes Grandpa was "good" and sometimes he was "bad." He explained that, since we didn't know when the "bad" behavior would occur, whatever medication we used would have to be given all the time. He prescribed a tranquilizing drug, and I began giving Grandpa one of the pills daily. It was hard to know whether the drug was doing any good. There was still "bad" behavior. Grandpa hadn't changed. I took him back to this doctor one more time, on the advice of a friend, to see if an injection of vitamin B would help. The doctor stated that he had no reason to believe it would help Grandpa, but since it wouldn't hurt him, he willingly administered the injection. Still no change occurred. I continued to give Grandpa the tranquilizer, experimenting with using two pills at particularly difficult times. I was still not convinced that it made any difference whatsoever.

Another topic discussed at the support group was bathing. We had been having problems with Grandpa's weekly shower, which Milt managed after dinner on Friday, Saturday, or Sunday evening. Grandpa was putting up a lot of resistance—refusing to go upstairs, refusing to take his clothes off, fighting with Milt over having to go into the shower. Milt couldn't handle refusal very well, and the situation was at a point where I was afraid Grandpa was going to fall and really get hurt. Someone at ADRDA suggested changing the time for his shower from evening to morning. Again, a simple change. Morning was clearly Grandpa's best time of the day, so this made a big difference. Generally this worked out well, with only occasional outbursts of temper and noncooperation. The shower experience was a time of closeness between Milt and his father. As they worked together and touched one another, Grandpa seemed to have a sense of being loved by his son.

Milt and I worked together to carry out the entire project. I was good at getting Grandpa to follow me, so it was my job to escort him upstairs.

"C'mon, Grandpa, I want you to come with me."

"Yeah? Where to?"

"Come, I'll show you." I would walk slowly from the kitchen to the stairway leading to the bedrooms. Then I would step up on each stair slowly, while Grandpa grasped the handrail and followed right behind me. (This way he couldn't see how far he had to go.) At the top of the stairs, I would reach for his hand and guide him straight ahead. If he were in a disagreeable mood, he might stop at any point and refuse to continue. Usually, though, we would proceed to the bedroom, where I would say, "I need your shirt, Grandpa, so I can wash it. Let's take it off." I would begin unbuttoning, and he would help. He would have trouble getting the sleeves open. We would get the shirt off. "Okay, thank you. Now the pants. I have to wash them, too." We would proceed to the underwear and socks. I would put his shirt over his shoulders again so he wouldn't feel chilled. Meanwhile, Milt would be undressed and running the shower water in the adjoining bathroom. "Okay, Milt," I would say, and he would take Grandpa by the hand and lead him to the shower, where he had to step over the threshold and then sit on a high stool with his back to the stream of water. It was always a shock at first.

"Too cold!"

"How's that, dad, okay?"

"I don't need that."

"Yes, you do. Doesn't if feel good?"

"Yeah, I guess so."

"Here, wash your arms with this." Milt would hand him a well-lathered washcloth. Grandpa would obey dutifully and hand it back. More lathering. "Now your legs." Grandpa would bend down from his sitting position to wash his legs. Milt would wash his feet. "Now your chest." And so on. Milt would have him stand to wash between his legs. When he was all scrubbed, Grandpa would have to turn around and sit again so that Milt could wash his hair. "Now, Dad, hold the washcloth over your eyes like this, okay?"

I would stay nearby so that I could lend a hand when and if Grandpa balked at any point. If he did, it was usually at the shampoo. The shower finished, Milt would help Grandpa to dry himself and then step on the bathroom scale so that he could record his weight. Then he would splash a little cologne on him.

"Oh, my, what's that for? I don't get next to no women!"

"Well, you never know, Dad. Scout's motto: Be Prepared!" It was their little joke.

I would have Grandpa's clean clothes all laid out on the bed, and Milt would give him one item at a time to put on. The socks were too hard for him because he couldn't straighten his ankles, but he insisted on doing as much as he could. Then they would go back downstairs.

"Wow, Grandpa, you look good," I would say to him. He would beam a big smile.

"Are you going dancing tonight, Grandpa?" Mike would tease. "I bet you're going to see your girlfriend!"

"Maybe," he winked at me. "I used to dance, years ago. . . . I used to dance with the ladies. . . . Not no more. You know, sometimes I think I find a woman. . . . get married. . . . But I'm afraid. . . . No, I'm too old. That's for you young folks." There had been a widow who was pursuing him at one point, but he was afraid she was after his money.

Grandpa clung to his unpredictability. There were still times when he put up such a fuss that we had to give up showering him until another day. There were also times when it was too late in the process to quit, and we had to fight him—literally—to finish the job. Grandpa was a fighter, and he had great strength in his arms, especially when it came to something he didn't want to do.

Some families are embarrassed by their Alzheimer's patients who remove all their clothes at inappropriate times. Grandpa had no such inclination, but he did have a fascination for shoes, items that were easy to encounter in our house. We had stressed "no shoes on the carpet" after purchasing new carpeting for the living room and stairway years ago, and the children had formed the habit of kicking their shoes off by the door—and leaving them there. Also, there were the extra shoes: gardening shoes, galoshes, house slippers, sneakers in good condition, sneakers with worn-out toes. We kept a rack for these various shoes which became Grandpa's "toy box." He would take off one or both of his shoes and put on one or both of someone's two-sizes-larger, bright green and white sneakers. Or try to put on someone's two-sizes-smaller, bright blue sneakers. When he succeeded and walked around in these oddly bright-colored shoes, it looked incongruous with his drab, baggy pants, his plaid flannel shirt, and his cap perched jauntily on his head—it was quite funny.

But when the owner of these shoes came to find them in a rush to go somewhere, it wasn't quite so funny.

Many families have their mythical "Mr. Nobody" who causes mischief by losing things. For us, Grandpa was the elf who got blamed for all sorts of missing objects. Sometimes a long-lost article would be found, in midsummer, in the pocket of Grandpa's winter coat. Occasionally Grandpa, who had never moved very fast in his entire life, hid something in the blink of an eye—or so it seemed, because he would find the least likely places to hide things, for instance, in a flower-pot under the leaves of the plant, or behind the toilet tank, or deep in his clothes closet. The very first place we went to look for things was in his dresser drawers, which contained a complete disarray of old underwear interspersed with Grandpa's treasures: string wrapped around a roll of paper, rubber bands, torn photos, and pages from magazines and books. Of course, we also blamed Grandpa for taking many things that eventually turned up right where we had misplaced them ourselves.

In the fall of Grandpa's third year with us, our Couples' Discussion Club, a group of people from church who met monthly in members' homes, had elected to use a booklet called *New Testament Way to Community*, by Desmond O'Donnell, OMI. The content was such that we divided into groups of five or six people to ponder some brief Scripture readings on a theme and then respond to questions of a personal and sharing nature. I found myself so immersed in the care of Grandpa that I responded to almost all questions from that perspective. I began to realize that this was the most profound experience of my life, and that my sharing of the insights I had gained helped others to share theirs also.

One session delved into personhood and God's love for each

of us, which created in each person a need to love and to be loved. The sharing that took place was both touchingly beautiful and sad, as it revealed the different perceptions of people in the group and the love or lack of love that they had experienced in their lives.

That night I must have dreamed about the session, because I awoke early in the morning with a powerfully warm sense of God's presence in my life and his abiding love. I lay there for a while, just enjoying this sensation. The words of Mary's canticle (Luke 1:46–55) from the Bible began going through my mind, only it wasn't Mary's song, it was my own. I reached for my notebook and recorded my thoughts in a poem which I called "My Magnificat" or "My Song of Joy." It was a "mountain-top" experience for me.

My Magnificat

My soul rejoices in the Lord who created me,
My being sings praise to God, my Savior.
For the Lord, the most holy one, has loved me!
He has seen this lowly handmaiden
    and has done many things for me.
Holy is his name.
He has fashioned me with his very hand
    all the days of my life.
My family, my friends, my talents,
    everything I am,
In his wisdom he gave me.
Hills to climb, skies dark with night,
    wondrous dawns he has given me.
The miracle of life in my womb he gave me,
And his children to nourish and love,
Waking me to learn more of him.
Gifts too numerous to count he made mine.
Gently he knocked at my heart.
I had only to look for him, to acknowledge him,
And his gift of love has overflowed in me.
Wonderful is my God, the Creator of the Universe!
Glory and Praise be his forevermore!

Fall tuned to winter, bringing the anticipation of family holidays. Traditionally, Thanksgiving had been my time to host my side of the family. This year was no exception. There were sixteen of us around the table, including my sisters Betty and Pat and some old and dear friends. Our daughter Marian and her fiancé Jim, who had just become engaged, were eating dinner with Jim's family and would arrive later that evening. In spite of the crowd and the hustle-bustle of entertaining, Grandpa took it all in stride, most likely because there was always one person paying attention to him. My sister Betty was great at that. While everyone sat around sluggishly after the overabundant meal, I assigned them a few questions, for example: What animal would you like to be? and What is your earliest pleasant memory? I like to spring things like this as a little challenge. It was good. There were some chuckles, some old stories retold. Everyone had a chance to participate. Grandpa interrupted a few times until Milt invited him to go to bed, and he did. Cindy was bored. She would have preferred some more active games like those we had played in other years. It was, however, a very satisfying day.

Christmas saw the continuation of some other traditions. We had picked names, and everyone bought or made just one gift for our Christmas exchange. This custom had started when Marian was in college and had gone through various revisions till it reached its present state. It made Christmas less materialistic and much less hectic for all of us.

A new tradition that had started since Grandpa had been living with us was visiting the Pinewood Nursing Home, the home where he had spent a pleasant two weeks during his first summer with us, on Christmas day. The previous Christmas, we had asked the director ahead of time for permission to sing carols to the residents. Many of them were out visiting with their families that day, but others were confined to the home and were glad to have us come. It was an effort to reach out beyond ourselves in some way, Grandpa's plight having made all of our children more sensitive to the needs of the elderly. Now a vote was taken, and it was agreed that we would go again this year. Our daughter Pat suggested that we make some little gifts to give to the residents. Being a teacher of small children, she had lots of ideas for simple crafts. So she invited all of her siblings to her and John's home on Christmas Eve for dinner and to spend the night. They would make the little gifts—simple Christmas ornaments—while watching *It's a Wonderful Life*, the Jimmy Stewart movie classic, on television. A new tradition—the "Christmas Eve sibling party"—was born.

Milt and I spent Christmas Eve feverishly finishing a wall-papering project upstairs in our bedroom, while making many trips downstairs to minister to Grandpa. Fortunately he went to bed early, and after the last strip was hung, Milt gathered the debris while I cooked a steak dinner for the two of us. We added wine and candlelight. At eleven we walked to Midnight Mass, leaving Grandpa asleep.

On Christmas morning, Grandpa woke up early but was easily satisfied so we could doze a couple of hours longer. After breakfast Milt helped me with dinner preparations. From one of his teachers, he had obtained a pattern for small banners that he and I could make for the nursing home residents; we put together ten or so of them, feeling good that we would have something of our own to share.

Marian and Jim, who had attended Jim's family's party instead of the "sibling party," arrived at two o'clock followed by the rest of the family, and shortly thereafter we all piled into several cars, Grandpa too, and were en route to the nursing home. Another family, friends of ours, joined us there. We marched rather hesitantly through the halls, clutching our carol songbooks as we sang, making up with enthusiasm what was lacking in musical quality. Seeing the faces of these residents, their haggard expressions and wan smiles, choked me up. I had trouble singing at all. But Grandpa's voice boomed out. He knew "Jingle Bells" and "Silent Night," though his tempo was a little slow. Some of the residents sang along with us, too.

Pat distributed several of the handmade gifts to each of us, and it was up to us to hand them out. It wasn't easy to approach someone who looked so close to death itself and say, "Merry Christmas!" Cindy did it very graciously. She walked right up close and smiled warmly, touching each person gently as she spoke.

We stayed only one hour, then quickly made our exit and drove home. After dinner and our gift exchange, we piled into cars again for another traditional family gathering at the home of my sister Eileen and her family. This time Grandpa stayed home. He was already asleep, and Terese volunteered to stay with him.

Victims of Alzheimer's disease frequently respond to a challenge and "rise to the occasion," as they say. Grandpa surprised us on New Year's Day that year. It was his eighty-fifth birthday, reason enough for another traditional family gathering.

After dinner, when it was time for dessert, I brought the cake with lighted candles and set it before Grandpa as we all sang "Happy Birthday." He was overcome; tears came to his eyes. He stood and actually made a little speech! "Thank you. Thank you. There were times . . . I don't know how far back it was . . . I was all alone. Three, four days, all alone. . . . My wife, she was a good girl. . . . You people are so good. . . . Thank you. I could cry. . . . "

Indeed, there were other moist eyes in the room.

After the holidays, Milt and I talked about our vacation plans for the next summer, realizing that a family trip might not be possible this year. My phone calls to places that advertised "respite care" proved disappointing. These homes would not take anyone with serious problems (Grandpa's behavior being a serious problem).

For the first time in our marriage, Milt and I planned to take separate vacations. I would return to Green Lake for one week at the Christian Writers' Conference in August. Milt found a friend who was interested in backpacking. They made arrangements to go to the Upper Peninsula of Michigan for one week during July. We would not need an outside person to take care of Grandpa.

As the weeks and months wore on, however, maintaining our equanimity under the stress of caring for Grandpa continued to be difficult. Our constant feelings of frustration easily erupted in anger.

It was a Friday, my customary day to do the weekly house cleaning. Grandpa had been more annoying than usual, calling me constantly, accusing me of taking his money, complaining of having nothing to eat although he had been eating continually. I had finally finished cleaning the bathrooms and started dusting the furniture in the dining and living rooms.

Grandpa sat at the kitchen table. He had just eaten a slice of bread with applesauce. Now he looked dejected, depressed.

"What's the use?" he said. "I don't want to live. Nothing. I ain't got nothing." He sat with arms hanging loose at his sides, head down, eye lids drooping and nearly closed. As I walked near him, I could tell he was following me with his eyes. He seemed to be watching to make sure I got the effect.

"What's the matter, Grandpa?" I asked.

"All alone. My dear wife, she passed away. I took good care of her. I don't know why, now I'm all alone." He shook his head sadly from side to side.

Feeling sorry for him, I sat and held his hand for a while, then tried to interest him in some pictures. He seemed to feel better, so I went back to my work.

"You don't care," he said, returning to his depressed attitude. "Nothing. They don't give me nothing. I'm going." He got up and began shuffling toward the door.

I didn't feel like chasing after him, so I hurried past him, got the key, threw the deadbolt into place, returned the key to its hiding place, and went back to my cleaning.

He tried to open the door. "Open!" he shouted. "I want to get out! Let me out!"

"Grandpa, I'm sorry, I can't let you go right now. I'm trying to get some work done. You can come here and work. Come on, I'll show you."

"No! Out, I want out! Bastar's, that's what you are! You're no good!"

"It does no good to try to be nice to him," I thought to myself. "He's just too demanding." I remembered his constant calls for attention all morning, his restlessness, his insatiable appetite, his moodiness. He was never satisfied. How could I get anything done? I was feeling pressure because some friends were coming over that evening.

Grandpa was still angry, walking around shouting his insults. I ignored him. I went to the broom closet, got out the vacuum cleaner and the attachment I needed, and started over to the stairway to the second floor. He followed me. I plugged in the cord, then picked up the tank and started upstairs with it.

"No!" he shouted. "Don't do that! Come back here!"

I couldn't believe it. He started up the stairs after me and grabbed the hose. We stood there engaged in a tug-of-war for the vacuum cleaner! All the time he was shouting insults and calling me names, his eyes glaring at me.

My blood began to boil. I could feel my face flushing with anger. The thought that I could push him down the stairs flashed through my mind. I jerked the hose to one side to throw him off balance. He was holding onto the railing with one hand or he surely would have fallen.

With a look of surprise and fear, he backed down the stairs slowly, relinquishing his grip on the hose.

"You son of a bitch! You're no good. I hate you!" He kept shouting the same words over and over.

For a moment I stood, hating him, wishing I'd had the nerve to make him fall. My arms were shaking with the surge of emotion that filled me.

I descended the stairs, set the vacuum cleaner down, went around to the basement door, and walked down the basement stairs, closing the door behind me. I had to get away from him.

Downstairs I sat in the semidarkness, feeling my whole body shaking with rage. For some moments I just sat, not conscious of any thought, until the tremors ceased.

Gradually, a feeling of shame and remorse came over me. "Lord, forgive me!" I prayed. What had happened to me that I had so completely lost my temper? I thought about Grandpa. What if he had fallen and been seriously hurt?

I took some deep breaths, slowly gaining control of myself. I still felt shaky, unsure, remorseful. "Lord, give me peace," I prayed. "Forgive me for wanting to hurt Grandpa. Help me, Lord! I need you. I can't do this alone!"

I tried to reconstruct what had happened, to uncover some reason for Grandpa's behavior. Maybe he thought I was taking something that belonged to him, stealing it and going away with it. His first thought had been to grab it back. That must have been it! If I had tried to talk to him, I would have known; none of this would have happened.

For a few minutes longer I sat, mindful of how wrong I had been in allowing my irritation with Grandpa to build up into an explosion of anger. "The man is crazy," I told myself. "He does and says things that make sense only in his strange inner world. I cannot let his behavior influence my own. I am caring for him because he needs me. I do it freely. This is life's challenge for me right now, and my response to it determines my growth, or lack of it." I sighed a deep sigh of relief, feeling as if a weight had been lifted. Tears began flowing down my cheeks, soothing healing tears.

"Thank you, Lord! Thank you for this opportunity for me to see myself more clearly. Thank you for the strength to carry on!"

Finally I went upstairs, a little embarrassed, and hesitant to face Grandpa. He was sitting at the table arranging his papers.

"The lady is mad at me," he said.

"It's all right now, Grandpa. I'm sorry. I'm not mad anymore." I fixed him another slice of bread and applesauce and went back to my vacuum cleaning. Another crisis had passed.

Subsequently a biography of Mother Teresa of Calcutta happened to come to my attention. I read it and was struck by her life of unconditional love of the most rejected of human beings. She wrote a little prayer, "Though you hide yourself behind the unattractive disguise of the irritable, the exacting, the unreasonable, may I still recognize you and say, Jesus, my patient, how sweet it is to serve you."* I copied it and put it on my refrigerator door so that I would remember to read it often. Another book was suggested to me: *The Art of Loving* by Eric Fromm.† Fromm described the devastating results of loneliness and made me conscious of Grandpa's need to be with people.

One brisk Sunday afternoon in early spring, Milt decided to work outside in the yard and I joined him, bundling Grandpa up

*Malcolm Muggeridge, *Something Beautiful for God: Mother Teresa of Calcutta* (New York: Harper and Row, 1971), p. 75.
†Eric Fromm, *The Art of Loving* (New York: Harper and Row, 1974).

also for some fresh air. I raked leaves and dead grass while Milt trimmed dead branches from the trees and cut back the evergreens. Grandpa helped by picking up the cut branches and twigs and putting them into the garbage cans. Cindy came out, also, for a break from her piano practice.

Perhaps Grandpa became tired of his job or thought it was time to "go home." Anyway, he began walking down the sidewalk. Cindy followed beside him, while Milt and I continued our yard work. They walked to the end of the block and turned north. After quite some time elapsed and Cindy and Grandpa didn't come back, I called Terese, who was doing schoolwork upstairs, and asked if she would hop on her bike and see where they were. She did so, and soon came back to report that they were six or seven blocks away and still going further. "Grandpa doesn't want to come back. Cindy wants to know what she should do."

After more time had elapsed and another bicycle reconnaissance was made, we realized that Grandpa had walked farther than he had ever walked since he had lived with us, and that he probably wouldn't be able to walk back, even if he wanted to. Milt got in the car and located the two of them, Cindy still patiently walking beside Grandpa, who shuffled along inches at a step. By this time, he was tired enough to appreciate a ride. He accepted the offer and returned home in the car, obviously fatigued from the exertion. What had impelled him to walk away? We would never know.

That night Milt helped Grandpa to get ready for bed. They made the trip to the bathroom and to the bedroom, where Grandpa untied his shoes and took them off. Then he lay back on his pillow while Milt held his hand for a few moments. Milt was surprised when Grandpa said, "You're so good. I love you." Milt had a strong feeling that Grandpa knew he was speaking to his son when he said these words—words that Milt had longed to hear as a young boy. It had taken a long time, but Milt was glad that his dad had finally been able to express his affection verbally, and that he, Milt, had made it possible by having Grandpa at home with us. There were a few other times when Grandpa said "I love you" to Milt during the next few months, at times when they had close moments together. It seemed that

Grandpa was aware that he was gradually failing. These expressions of love meant a lot to Milt. Later he would describe them as a high point in the experience of caring for his dad. If Grandpa had been in a nursing home for all this time, Milt might have missed the opportunity to hear those words of love. They might have remained unspoken.

7 · The Fourth Year

One evening in May, during Grandpa's fourth year with us, Milt and I left the house at seven o'clock, with assurance from Terese and Cindy that they would watch Grandpa. We were team-teaching an eight-week course called "Discovering the Bible" at our church. It was easy for me to find myself volunteering to do things like this. There was a need for such programs, and neither of our priest-associates at that particular time had the interest or the time to do them. It was I who had made the commitment. Milt had agreed to be there, help me, and give moral support, while I would organize the class and do the necessary preparation, using a manual that made it easy. I knew that getting out on Thursday evenings for eight weeks would present difficulties, but I figured I'd find some way to do it.

That evening, Terese and Cindy were both at home, and they agreed to take turns with Grandpa. He had gone to bed readily and seemed to be settled for the night, so they went upstairs to their bedrooms to do their schoolwork. Grandpa usually called out if he wanted attention or if he couldn't sleep, but he was silent. The front door was not bolted, and they didn't hear it open. He didn't announce, "I'm going!" as he often did. He just left quietly. Some time later, Mike came home and noticed Grandpa's bedroom door open and his bed empty. He went upstairs, thinking that Grandpa might be up there with Terese. "Where's Grandpa?" he asked.

"In bed."

"No, he's not."

"Oh, my gosh! Did he go out? I didn't hear anything!"

"Terese! How could you forget about him?" Mike ran downstairs.

Cindy heard the commotion. "Did Grandpa run away? I didn't hear him!"

They both ran down the stairs as Mike was going out the front door. "What shall we do?" they called after him.

"I don't care!" he flung out angrily as he dashed down the street.

"What'll we do?" Cindy asked again, as the two girls stood in the open doorway.

"Mike'll find him. I'm going to finish my chemistry." Although at other times Terese was very concerned about Grandpa, her schoolwork was more compelling at the moment.

"Maybe we should go look for him, too."

But they didn't. When Milt and I returned at nine-thirty, the two girls reported what had happened, apologizing for their oversight.

Milt and I got into the car and drove around slowly, peering frantically up and down the dark sidewalks, thinking of all kinds of misfortunes that could have befallen Grandpa, and wondering whether Mike had found him. I remembered that someone at the support group had shared information about identification bracelets for just such an eventuality, and I upbraided myself for neglecting to order one for Grandpa.

Finally Milt drove through a main intersection which is located three or four blocks from our house, where a plaza with a number of small stores, banks, and a gas station with bright lights illuminated the warm spring night. There on a bench beside a Burger King restaurant sat two figures which turned out to be Grandpa and Mike.

They sat, talking calmly, quietly, Mike vainly trying to persuade Grandpa to walk home. Mike had found him wandering and had walked with him until he spied the bench and pointed it out to Grandpa, who knew enough to seek a place to sit down. Now he wouldn't budge. He was holding a grapefruit in each hand. They had been in his large pants pockets, and he didn't know what they were or "who put them there." After we spent five or ten more minutes trying to get him to come with us,

Grandpa finally got up and walked slowly to where our car was parked. For about two hours he had been agitated, unpersuadable, refusing to cooperate in returning home.

The next evening, the supper dishes were still on the table when the doorbell rang and a friend of Mike's came in with her young nephew. Mike and Terese rushed off to get their camping gear for the weekend trip they had planned to take with these friends. They began making trips up and down the stairs, in and out to the car with their duffle bags and boxes of supplies. In the midst of this bustle of activity, Grandpa decided to leave. Milt intercepted him. A violent struggle ensued, the two of them engaged in a wrestling match and shouting loud epithets at each other. Grandpa's anger gave him a surge of strength in his arms and a viselike grip in his hands. Milt, in turn, refused to give up the contest. In the scuffle, the fragile outer layer of skin on Grandpa's wrist was torn, and several drops of blood oozed out and appeared on the floor. Milt, contrite at seeing this, called for a Band-Aid. It took two of us to get the bandage in place.

Long after Mike and Terese had left with their friends, Grandpa remained highly agitated and restless. At nine o'clock he finally went to bed and was quiet for the night.

At lunchtime on the following day, a Saturday, Cindy's friend Krista came to play. Grandpa reacted almost immediately, becoming upset and telling Krista to go home. The two girls put up with this abuse just as long as they had to, and then went outside to play ball. Grandpa was not appeased. He followed them outside and shouted to Krista, "You go home, you hear? Go home! I'll shoot you! Get out of here!" When Milt and I tried to get him to let the girls alone and come back inside, he turned his fury on me and said, "You bastar'! I'll kill you. Get away from me!" We got him into the house, but it was quite a while before he calmed down. Milt gave him a glass of wine. I put out a dish of applesauce and some graham crackers. In all, this latest "attack" lasted two hours.

Three incidents of what might be termed "catastrophic reactions" had occurred in three days!* Attacks like this had never

---

*I was not familiar at that time with Nancy L. Mace and Peter V. Rabins, M.D., *The 36-Hour Day: A Family Guide to Caring for Persons with Alzheimer's Disease,* been so frequent before. What was going on with Grandpa? Was he entering a new phase?

Grandpa's insistence on leaving seemed to me to be his way of solving his problems—his loneliness, confusion, desire for some unattainable something that would make things better for him. Perhaps it was an unconscious need to return to the past. Whatever the cause, it was something he couldn't help.

Grandpa's problem behavior occurred at various times. Sometimes it was provoked by a family situation, such as the bustle of activity in preparation for the camping trip. Other times it happened when Grandpa was completely alone and quiet, perhaps the victim of his own thoughts. Still other occasions seemed to be provoked by our attempt to coerce Grandpa into doing something he didn't want to do, or conversely, by an attempt to stop him from doing something he wanted to do. To prevent these "attacks" or "catastrophic reactions," we tried to keep a calm atmosphere, refused to argue with Grandpa when we could avoid it, let him have his way whenever possible, gave him simple instructions and plenty of time to respond, and spent time with him to ease his loneliness. All these measures helped to minimize the volatile upsets that were so disruptive to our daily need for peace.

Yet it did seem that we were seeing a new phase—a change in Grandpa's behavior that necessitated a new response, perhaps, or at least a deeper reach into our resources for patience and acceptance of Grandpa and this strange disease.

What were Terese's and Cindy's reactions to all of this? I wish I could say that Milt and I sat down and asked them about their feelings and thoughts or gave them a chance to respond to what was going on. Unfortunately, we were so caught up in our own response—attempting to prevent this behavior in Grandpa if possible—that we failed to consider what impact his behavior might have on our young daughters. They were aware that Grandpa

---

Related Dementing Illnesses, and Memory Loss in Later Life (Baltimore: Johns Hopkins University Press, 1982), but it describes this overreacting on pages 25–26: "People with brain diseases often become excessively upset and may experience rapidly changing moods. Strange situations, confusion, groups of people, noises, being asked several questions at once, or being asked to do a task that is difficult for them can precipitate these reactions."

had a brain disease and couldn't help being the way he was, but Grandpa had used threatening words during his outburst this time. We never discussed any possible fears the girls may have had. We had never taken Grandpa's words very seriously, so the threats were dismissed from our minds with all the rest. I made a greater effort to have a sitter here during our evening classes so that the responsibility for Grandpa would not be thrust onto the children.

Paid sitters had not worked out before, but Grandpa had changed. He might be less resistant to a stranger now. I called the church rectory on the chance that they might have the names of some people who were willing to care for the elderly on a sporadic, part-time basis.

The time was right. There were two women who would care for elderly people. I called them. One agreed to come on Thursday evenings for the duration of the Bible class. After that, I continued to call upon each of them several times each month, either in the daytime or evening. Grandpa gradually became used to them, and they accepted his occasional outbursts of temper and hostile behavior.

Meanwhile, there were other things going on that were important also. On June 11, Cindy would graduate from eighth grade; on the evening after, Terese would graduate from high school—and two days later their eldest sister would be married! (Why is it that family activities have a way of bunching up like that?)

Marian's wedding was the main event for all of us, superseding graduation celebrations. Both Terese and Cindy were bridesmaids (Cindy a junior bridesmaid, without a male partner). Both were caught up in the selection of dresses, the showers, the rehearsal, and all the other facets of the occasion. Pat was her sister's matron of honor. Mike and Mart were not in the wedding party but couldn't help catching some of the excitement.

Being twenty-six years old and having been independent for five years, Marian planned her own wedding, together with her fiancé, Jim. I had my hands full with Grandpa, so I was grateful not to get too involved. As the day approached, Marian was concerned about whether or not we would take Grandpa to the reception. She wanted him to be there, to be a part of it; she wanted him to be in the photographs, as he had been when Pat had been married three years earlier. But he had become so much more disoriented and easily riled that I couldn't permit it. I didn't want the celebration to be spoiled for me or anyone else by Grandpa's presence. Crowds were too unsettling for him. It would be better if we could have him taken care of somehow.

My friend Mary from RE:AL agreed to have Grandpa at her home for the entire day. Marian still wanted to go there in her wedding dress and have a picture taken, but in the end she dropped the idea. Grandpa would not have understood and would not remember it anyway.

The day came with a light morning shower giving way to sunshine. Grandpa was safely dispatched to Mary's home with a word of caution about his use of the bathroom. Recently he had been missing the stool and wetting the floor. Mary understood and promptly pulled up the carpet from her bathroom floor. By now Grandpa accepted her easily and did not make any fuss when I left without him.

The lovely wedding ceremony brought tears of joy to my eyes. Afterward quite a number of people accepted the invitation to come to our home, since there was a delay of several hours before the evening reception. I had opted for an easy solution to entertaining the group, hiring two women who brought hors d'oeuvres and all necessary supplies and graciously served our guests. It was one party I thoroughly enjoyed.

Nothing solidifies a family quite so much as a wedding. All the children entered into the exhilaration of the day, and music and dancing rounded out the evening. Mart surprised us with his own special attire: a vintage white silk shirt, bow tie, pleated tweed trousers—all purchased from a thrift store—and some black oriental slippers. His long hair was tied back in a ponytail in the style of Thomas Jefferson. He was a totally free spirit, enjoying himself without a sip of alcoholic drink, and his new-found exuberance spilled over to Terese and Cindy as they danced and let go of shyness and inhibitions to laugh and make merry. It was good to see them having such a good time together.

Grandpa spent the day much as he would have at home. He

and Mary sat outside and watched the birds and the neighborhood children at play. After lunch she suggested a walk, so they started around the block. This was the wrong thing to do, Mary said, because Grandpa decided to go home. "Lady, you go on. I'll go myself," he told her. She was having some difficulty with him, and his loud voice alerted the neighbors, who came out to ask what the trouble was. Mary explained briefly and continued on. Grandpa walked quite a distance, Mary trailing him all the way. Then, unexpectedly, when she caught up with him he was happy to see her and accepted her offer to go and have a drink. (She carefully avoided using the word "home," she said.) They walked back together.

When they arrived at Mary's house, Grandpa insisted on carrying the lawn chairs into the house and rearranging the living room furniture to make room for them. Mary let him have his way.

In late afternoon Grandpa started getting restless to leave, but he was persuaded to wait until after dinner. Mary's husband, Jerry, tried to talk to him about baseball and other topics but didn't get very far with it. He found it hard to understand what was wrong with Grandpa.

After dinner Mary invited Grandpa to go for a ride in the car, and Mary and Jerry brought Grandpa to our house, which was now empty because all of us were at the reception. "This is just like my house," Grandpa exclaimed as he walked around into the various rooms. He was reluctant to go to bed at first, but eventually he conceded that he was tired. He wouldn't let Mary take his shoes off; he did it himself, then lay down on the bed and was soon asleep. I had arranged for a teenage son of some good friends to come and stay with Grandpa at this point, so Mary and Jerry could go home. Grandpa slept peacefully until morning, when we were all back and ready to face a new day.

And so summer began. Terese had already found a new part-time job, working at the Pinewood Nursing Home, where Grandpa had stayed for two weeks during his first summer with us, and where we had gone as a family to sing carols on Christmas Day. The work was demanding and difficult but also rewarding. Terese became good friends with some of the residents, but there were others she "couldn't stand" and didn't like taking care of. It was a good experience for her, and she knew it. In July she and Milt drove some 200 miles to Macomb, Illinois, where Terese registered as a freshman at Western Illinois University, beginning a new period in her life.

Also in July, Milt and his friend Ray traveled to the Porcupine Mountains of Michigan for their first real backpacking experience. They withstood the rigors of rain and insects and returned refreshed, convinced that desolate, uninhabited areas have a beauty that can best be appreciated in no other way than backpacking.

Cindy spent a quiet summer enjoying her own pursuits: piano, guitar, dance lessons, and numerous library books to read. She also kept a diary. Much later, for the writing of this book, she shared some passages with me.

> Franta (the dreaded one) is getting more uptight every day.* I wish I could say that I love him, but those times are few and far between. Almost everything I do in his presence he has a fit about. All the time he's yelling at me, I'm muttering under my breath that I hate him. I even tried making up a terrible song about how I'd like to kill him. I know it's terrible. I hate to even write it down. I know I would not even try to kill or hurt him. Sometimes I'd like to hug and kiss him.

And another day:

> I took care of my grandfather all afternoon today. It's strange, but I didn't mind being with him. I even had fun. We played a game where we kicked Superballs with our feet in the foyer. He played sitting down. There was another downpour this afternoon. I watched it with Franta. After it died down a lot, I jumped in the puddles to amuse him.

I regret that I didn't encourage Cindy to express these feelings to me at the time.

---

*Franta is a pet name, meaning Frank, in Bohemian.

Mike, at twenty-four, expressed his feelings by way of complaints about being "stuck" at home, predicting that he was going to move out but finding no way to do so. His summer activities included a job at the "Y" as a day camp counselor and his volunteer work with church youth groups, a movement that area Catholic churches had recently become involved in. Mart, on the other hand, was in northern Wisconsin, also working as a "Y" camp counselor for the summer, with no plans for the future except to continue making Wisconsin his home. He had dropped out of college for the time being.

Soon it was August and my turn to be away from home. A week at Green Lake reaffirmed me in spirit. My poetry class and instructor inspired me to devote more time to writing, if I could find a way to give it some priority in my life.

As fall approached, Grandpa's escapades continued, not every day but with increasing frequency. He resisted going to bed in the evening, so that many times it was eight, nine, or ten o'clock and he was still up, prowling restlessly around the house or demanding to go outside. We would often give him a glass of wine, hoping that if the tranquilizer didn't help to relax him, the alcohol would. Nothing changed, unless it gradually worsened.

One October morning, Grandpa had been alone in the family room for some time after he finished his breakfast. I was occupied with various things—my morning meditation, putting on my make-up, bed making, and laundry. Mike came home from his morning bus route. Grandpa was wrapping things in paper and stuffing his pockets.

The phone rang. It was my friend Mary, whom I had asked to take care of Grandpa for us again. Milt had been invited to make a presentation at a principals' conference in New Orleans in November. Since we had been unable to vacation together during the summer, he had invited me to accompany him on this four-day trip. Mary was calling to say that she had decided to take the job, and there were many details to discuss.

As we were about finished (or so I thought), Grandpa went outside. I saw Mike going to talk with him, and I mentioned to Mary that Grandpa had just "taken off," but that Mike was with him. We talked for perhaps five more minutes.

As soon as I was off the phone, I went out to the garage, which was open, and called. Mike was not there. Then I saw him running toward me from the corner, carrying Grandpa's coat.

"I couldn't find him," he said. "I persuaded him to come back once, but I turned my back and he was gone again."

I got my car keys and hopped into the car. As I pulled out, I saw Mike starting his car also. I cruised slowly through a four- or five-block area to the east, then drove through an area to the west.

Back on our street again, I saw that Mike's car was in front of the house. I pulled into the drive. "Did you find him?"

"I didn't see him," he said. So I backed out again, covering a slightly wider territory this time.

As I turned back east into a nearby busy street, I saw him, not more than a half block from home, but on the other side of the street. Evidently he had been talking to some man in his backyard, which is why we hadn't seen him earlier.

Grandpa would not get into my car. He would not go home, but I did get him to put on his coat. He would have nothing further to do with me and wanted me to go away. A policeman in a squad car slowed and had his window open, acting as if he were concerned. I asked him if my son had called. "Yes," he said, "Do you need help?" He pulled around in front of us. Grandpa was gruff with him and indicated to the policeman that he didn't know who I was and didn't trust me.

I assured the policeman that I would simply stay with Grandpa until he decided to go back home; so he left, saying he'd tell my son where we were.

Shortly after that, Mike came along, but Grandpa would have nothing to do with him either.

For the next hour, I walked with Grandpa in a brisk wind while he rang doorbells. He consistently refused to go back home and wanted to be rid of me. I left him and kept watch from a distance. Then Mike took his turn and finally succeeded in persuading him to go back. Grandpa threatened to leave home several more times that day while Mike was with him and I had left on an errand.

During this fourth year of his stay with us, Grandpa became

increasingly preoccupied with leaving, or "going home." By this time there were fewer activities that could engage his interest, so that at times during the day—some days more than others, some days not at all—he would become noticeably restless, walking around constantly, looking for "something" or "something to do."

As his restlessness and agitation increased, he would go to the door to look outside. If the weather was not inviting, he might close the door and walk away, only to be back again after a minute or two. This would continue for half an hour or so, and then he would go outside in spite of the rain, snow, or cold. Often he would go from the front door around to the back of the house, where I would greet him and invite him to come in. It was as if he had found the place he was looking for.

It was very helpful to have deadbolts on the doors so that Grandpa could not open them. Still, we wanted him to be free to go outside. Walking was good exercise for him. He often enjoyed walking around the yard or sitting in the sunshine, so normally the doors were unbolted. There was a carport at the front entrance where he would stand and get a taste of the weather.

"I'm going," he said one day as he bent over the table in the family room, gathering things to take with him: a cup and a saucer in one hand, a spoon and crumpled piece of paper thrust into his pocket. "All right. What's this?" He spoke to himself, taking things out of his pocket again, checking the other pocket, smoothing out the piece of paper, folding it up carefully, putting it back into the pocket with the spoon, talking all the while, sometimes Bohemian words, sometimes just mumbled sounds.

"I'm going," he said again, a note of determination in his voice.

"Where are you going, Grandpa?" I asked him.

"I'm going to my friends. I have friends out there. North. Or west. Over there." He gestured in the direction he usually headed when he decided to leave. "They're waiting for me."

"You can stay here, Grandpa. We're glad to have you stay." It was a weak attempt to dissuade him.

"No, they want me. I'm going." He took the cup and saucer with him, his body remaining bent as he walked. He inched toward the door and went outside with his shuffling gait, his arms swinging out from his sides as if to draw his body forward, the cap on his head giving him a jaunty appearance.

He stopped at the end of the driveway, paused to get his bearings, headed west. He looked like any other elderly gentleman as he walked along. Only the cup and saucer held in one hand seemed unusual.

At the corner he crossed the street and headed south, stopping to look both ways. I caught up with him and talked with him:

"Let's go back now, Grandpa."

"No, I'm going to my friends."

"Where are they?"

"Oh, they're up there. They're waiting for me. I haven't seen them for a long time."

"Do you know the address?"

"It's north. Or west. Oh, don't bother me. I'll find it. You go home."

I walked along with him, and he breathed audibly as he walked, stopping now and then to look at the unfamiliar homes. Each time he came to a driveway he hesitated, perhaps thinking it was a street.

Finally coming to the end of the short block, he headed west again, tiring visibly but seemingly propelled onward. At the next home he turned and shuffled to the door, rang the doorbell and waited, rang again.

"Grandpa, this is a stranger's house. You don't know these people." I prayed that there was no one at home.

"Never mind. I'm going to ask them." He knocked at the door, then walked to the garage and knocked on the big double door. No answer. Disappointed but undaunted, he started down the street again. After half an hour or more of this, I persuaded him to turn back and walk the long way home again.

I found it hard to accept this unreasonable behavior. Grandpa didn't have any friends living around here. How could he? I thought I could convince him of the absurdity by pointing out that he didn't know the addresses of these so-called friends. He rang doorbells anyway! Obviously he was not being rational. How could I expect a rational argument to convince him? But I did. It seemed so ridiculous to me. Furthermore, it put me in the uncomfortable position of looking foolish along with him—invading the privacy of strangers in this way.

Another afternoon began very quietly. While I was busy in the kitchen, Grandpa was alone in the family room "playing" with his papers—sheets torn from old catalogs, newspapers, junk mail. He was stuffing some into various pockets. Then he began to talk about "going." He took a saucer, his thick glass mug, and the plastic tumbler from the bathroom and started outside: back and around the house, then down the street.

Hearing him leave and allowing him to get a head start, I then trailed him to the end of the block and across the street. He changed direction from west to south. I joined him, and we talked about where he was going. He had some friends there. Where? He didn't know, but he'd find them. I should go home. The usual.

At the next block he turned west again and passed several more houses, ringing a doorbell at one of them and pounding on the garage. No one was home. He proceeded on his way.

A schoolgirl on a bike rode across the street in front of us and went around to the back of the next house. He called to her. "You! Little girl! Who is . . . What . . . My friend . . . Over there . . . "

She looked at him strangely and stopped her bike with one foot on the sidewalk, still staring at him with open mouth. I made a circular motion with my finger at my head indicating "he's mixed up," and she parked her bike at the rear and went into the house.

Grandpa followed her around to the back entrance! My heart sank. A woman came to the screen door but did not open it. He began speaking to her, again unable to express himself. "You know . . . How can I say . . . My friend . . . My, my . . . ." The woman stood there, waiting patiently without answering. She was obviously uncertain as to what this was about.

I explained that my father-in-law was very confused and was looking for some friends and did not want to go home.

"Well, I have to give a piano lesson now," she said.

"If you close the inside door he will understand. I'm sorry for the interruption."

"That's all right," she said. She closed the door firmly.

Then he went around to the front of the house and was going to ring the doorbell. Frantically, I convinced him that this was the same house, so he crossed the street and started down the next block. He rang another doorbell. A dog barked, but no one answered. Then he went around to the back of the house and knocked and called out, "Lady, anyone home?" several times.

He returned to the street and was continuing to walk on, when Mike rode up on his bike. Grandpa was so agitated by now that he didn't seem to recognize him. After some discussion, Grandpa said something about going "back home," so I told him that "back home" was the other way and got him to turn around to head back. After Mike left, we were walking along and some school-children came by. He called out to them in his gruff voice. They looked at him blankly, and a couple of them answered, "I don't know."

Then, to my dismay, he went around to the back door of the piano teacher's house again! Instead of following him, I sat in the shade of a tree (it was sunny and very warm). I wasn't sure how much more of this I could take. Grandpa stayed at the back of the house for what seemed like five minutes or more, calling, while I hoped that no one would hear or notice him. Finally I heard a lady's voice and went back to find that he was talking with a woman from the house behind this one. She was trying to explain to him that his "friend" was not home.

"He's with me," I said. "He's just confused and thinks there's someone here that he knows, but there isn't."

The woman nodded. "I see. I was just trying to explain to him that my neighbor is not at home. He was looking in the window and calling."

"Yes, I know. Thank you. C'mon, Grandpa. Let's go, now." He took my extended hand, and we walked slowly back to the sidewalk.

Tired by this time, he agreed to go back home with me and began protesting that it was too far. He followed along slowly, reluctantly, to the street. A car was parked there, a man and a little girl inside, waiting. He went over and asked the man whether it was his car. (Grandpa wanted a ride, although he did not say so.) I persuaded him to walk on. Should I go and get my car now? "No, darn it," I thought angrily, "he wanted to walk this far, let him walk back!" I was also hesitant to leave him. What would he do while I was gone? What would people think of me if he fell in the street or something? If Grandpa was confused, so was I.

We crossed the street, and another car pulled up right in front of us and drove into the garage that was close to the street. An older couple got out, and Grandpa began questioning them incoherently. They gave us a puzzled glance and walked into the house. Suddenly Grandpa looked at what he had in his hands (saucer, glass mug, and plastic cup) and said that something was missing. He was sure. "Maybe it's in your pocket," I said, just to humor him. He started to check his pocket, and in doing so he dropped the glass mug. It broke into a hundred pieces! I looked in the open garage for a broom and found one. Meanwhile, Grandpa began picking up the glass and cut his hand on it. The lady must have been observing us from the window, because she came out with a broom, dustpan, and garbage can and went back in for a Band-Aid. I offered thanks and apologies.

By the time we started on our way again, Grandpa was more tired than ever. We turned the corner and walked down a few feet while he muttered that I should get "one of those" (cars) and take him home.

Giving in at last, I left him and hurried home for the car. When I returned, he was talking to some more people—high-school age—and more explanation and persuasion was required before he agreed to get into the car.

By this time, I had had it with him! I wanted to go inside and forget him, but he would not let me out of his sight. Mike tried to talk to him; Grandpa, however, wanted to "finish it with the lady." I was tired, had a headache, and really felt like leaving for good myself. I gave him two tranquilizer pills and a snack, went to the sofa, and sank down, exhausted. Gradually, but very gradually, he calmed down.

*   *   *

Milt and I generally agreed that when Grandpa became agitated or "hyper" like this, we would let him go out and walk, at least to some extent, to expend his energy. (In retrospect, it may seem strange that we let him do this, but at the time it seemed to make sense.) However, we had different methods of handling his leaving. Mike had his method, too.

Mike's way was totally accepting. He just stayed with Grandpa no matter how far he went, constantly reassuring him and then suggesting, "You can go back, Grandpa, if you want to." Of course, Mike didn't have to do this very often.

My method was manipulative: "Let's go this way, Grandpa, this is where Honels live." "Let's turn around now, Grandpa, maybe you're getting tired."

Milt's method was most assertive: "You can't go across the street, Dad. Turn around." He would stand directly in front of Grandpa so there was no more walking until he turned around. This method might require half an hour or more of standing on the corner, blocking him from going in any direction except one: back home. It also involved some arm wrestling in the process.

Although generally I liked my own method of handling Grandpa, I found that Milt's method worked best for keeping Grandpa's wanderings within a reasonable range. I began to try it myself.

Living with Grandpa's tendency to "go home" was a constant test of control. Who had control? How much? Where to draw the line?

Following this old man with his slow, steady shuffle, arms swinging, one hand clutching his treasures as he headed resolutely down the street, provoked many unpleasant thoughts and feelings in me. Usually I was irritated to begin with, because I had been in the midst of preparing dinner or doing some other chore and had needed to drop everything to run after Grandpa. He was in control, I was not.

It was always uncertain when and how each escapade would end—how far would he walk, would he be too tired to walk back home again, how much of my time would be wasted, what if he fell or got hit by a car?

Then there was embarrassment, too. I didn't mind walking

along with Grandpa so much, but when he started ringing door-bells or going into people's yards, I was very uncomfortable.

Because his wandering happened so frequently, sometimes I would take my time about going after him, letting him get a head start. Then a neighbor would call and say, "Did you know Grandpa is down by so-and-so's?" I was glad for the concern, but it was a little embarrassing, too, because the neighbors might think I was not watching him carefully enough.

When this "hyper," agitated behavior came on, it seemed to me to be a physical/chemical impulse that propelled him. All his energy was focused on one objective: going away. No amount of reasoning made any difference. Yet he had enough sense left to know that turning around was going the wrong way. His body mechanism sometimes fought that to the point of dragging his feet, threatening to fall, and even falling—slowly, gently, on a soft, grassy spot. (Grandpa did this with me on a few occasions and created a whole new problem: how to get him up!)

Once this period of physical/chemical agitation had subsided—it would take an hour or two—then Grandpa was once more passive, usually hungry, and fairly content. Occasionally, though, he would start the whole process over again.

Often I just bolted the doors so Grandpa couldn't get out, but this was scary, too. When he discovered that he could not open the door, he fussed and fumed and banged on the door with his fist, cussing me out. I had to stay away from him until he calmed down, watching from a distance to make sure he didn't destroy anything of value. He never did, but listening to him frayed my nerves. I'd put some food out for him to find as he paced around. That sometimes distracted him. I used the bolted doors rather as a last resort: if he had already wandered once during the day, if I was doing something that I couldn't leave abruptly, or if the weather was inclement. I was always glad when, after I had been alone with Grandpa most of the day, Milt, Mike, or Cindy would come home. I felt the pressure leave me, as if steam had been building up in me and I needed someone else to be there, to take the lid off and dissipate that pressure. This was especially true on days when Grandpa had been particularly restless and de-manding, or hostile and "going home." When he headed down the street, I was never sure what he would do or how I'd get him back home again. I was thankful that when Milt was home, he took charge of Grandpa's wandering.

The house didn't seem quite the same, now that Terese was away at school. I didn't miss the loud blaring of rock music that accompanied her wherever she went, but now that she was away, I missed her especially in the kitchen. She loved to bake cookies and breads and conjured me into helping her. (I had my choice of whether to prepare the dry or the wet ingredients.) Terese had a way of wheedling anybody (even Grandpa) into doing anything she wanted, so that they had fun doing it.

Cindy noticed her absence, too. She missed Terese very much, because during the past year they had become friends as well as sisters. Now she had no one she wanted to confide in. "I feel like an only child! Why didn't you have more kids after me?" she demanded. There was nobody of her age. Mike was much too old to be friends with; her married sisters seemed more like aunts. Now she was a freshman in a huge high school where her friends from junior high were all dispersed, and she still had to use the map she had glued into the inside cover of her notebook so she could find her way to the next class.

Cindy turned to Grandpa as a fellow sufferer. She discovered that he liked it when she knelt by his chair and put her arm around his shoulder, leaning her head against him. He would sing for her. Sometimes they stood holding hands and swayed slowly to the rhythm as he sang. They were great balloon tossers, too, a game that Grandpa was very good at and seldom tired of playing.

College life, living in a dormitory, and being away from home and her close friends from high school—all hit Terese suddenly and hard. She suffered feelings of loneliness, evidenced by lengthy long-distance phone calls and complaints that a life that was 90% studying seemed terribly unbalanced. Gradually she made new friends, and the phone calls and letters we received became fewer and more positive in tone.

Mart was experiencing his own frustrations with life in Wisconsin. He had decided not to register for classes in September and to look for a job in Green Bay. This proved to be no easy task, however, as all he could find was a part-time paper route. He was fortunate in being able to live inexpensively with friends and to maintain a Spartan vegetarian lifestyle, supporting himself in part from his savings fund (for college) that he had earned during high school. We didn't hear from him very often, but suddenly, in early October, he announced that he was planning a long trip and needed to borrow a backpack. He would be heading north to Duluth, Minnesota, and then east to see what Canada was like, then traveling south as winter approached. He would hike or hitch rides, starting out with two friends and a dog—a black Labrador mixed breed he had procured as a protective measure.

We boxed and wrapped the backpack and sent it to him, and soon the three young people were on their way. The friends dropped out at various destinations, leaving Mart and his dog, Tsasha, to head southward alone. He phoned us at home every week or two, at our request, keeping us posted on his adventures. He reported that he would be in New Orleans in November at about the same time Milt and I would be there. We made plans to meet in front of our hotel, and so we did. Mart, in his ponytail and rugged camping attire, and Tsasha, on a chain, were standing and waiting for us as we pulled up in our cab from the airport.

Thanksgiving Day found a smaller group around our table. We all missed my lively sister Pat who had changed careers and moved to Houston in June. Mart was still not back from his trip. He had settled in Alabama temporarily, where he found a room with some college students and worked as a dishwasher in a restaurant. He would be home for Christmas, but he didn't know what he would do after that.

Soon it was Christmas Day. Dinner was over, gifts exchanged, Grandpa tucked in bed for the night (we hoped), and we sat around—just our family: ten of us, including Jim and John, our two sons-in-law. In the afternoon we had piled into three cars, Grandpa with us, for our annual brief visit to the Pinewood Nursing Home to sing Christmas carols to the people confined there on the holiday. Our daughter Pat (the schoolteacher) had again engineered a family crafts project, so that we had some small paper ornaments made from old Christmas cards as gifts for the elderly people. Mart didn't care to go with us. He stayed home and made eggnog.

Now we sat contentedly enjoying the rapport of family. The subject of the nursing home came up.

Marian: Cindy, I was amazed at how you went right up to those people and touched them and talked to them!

Cindy: Well, I . . . [shy smile].

Pat: I just couldn't do that. I didn't mind handing them the ornament, but I couldn't say any more than "Merry Christmas."

Rosalie: Neither could I. I couldn't even sing the carols. My voice kept choking up!

(*Shrieks of laughter*)

Pat: Mom! So did mine! Isn't that ridiculous?

Milt: No, it's not ridiculous. It means that you were very deeply touched by those people. That's good. You're sensitive.

Mike: Well, if you ever put Grandpa into a place like that, I'll . . .

Rosalie: You'll what, Mike? It's a very real possibility, so you'd better consider it.

(*Several voices all at once*)

Marian: Well, I think it's great that you're taking care of Grandpa. I couldn't do it. [*To Milt and Rosalie*] Don't you guys ever get that way!

Pat: John's parents had his grandmother at their house off and on. Then she had to go into a nursing home.

Rosalie: Yes, I remember that. She was kind of like Grandpa, wasn't she, John?

John: Yes, she acted funny, hiding things, wrapping things up in wads of paper, stuff like that.

Pat: And she stayed at your parents' house for a while, and then with your aunts and uncles, right?

John: Yeah, she spent a couple of months at each place, so it wasn't so hard. But then she got real bad and nobody could handle it, so they took her to a nursing home.

Rosalie: How long was she there? Do you remember?

John: A year, a couple of years, maybe. I'm not sure.

Terese: Well, I think you should keep Grandpa at home. Those people don't get good care. Some of them are just ignored a lot. [She spoke with inside knowledge, from her experience of the previous summer.]

Rosalie: Nursing homes are so expensive, too.

Several voices: How much does it cost?

Rosalie: A couple of thousand dollars a month, depending on how much care the person needs.

Cindy: Two thousand dollars a month? Wow!

Milt: Yes, but if they can't pay it, the state pays it.

Marian—the social worker: Dad! I hope you're not thinking of putting Grandpa on state aid! That's terrible!

Milt: No one said that. But if we did have to put Grandpa into a nursing home, how would we pay that kind of money?

Marian: Why don't you sell his house? [She and Jim, newly married, were living there and taking care of it for us.]

Milt: The house is in my name now and if we sell it, I'll divide the proceeds among you six kids. That's what Babi and Grandpa always wanted.

Marian: As far as I'm concerned, I don't want it. It should go to Grandpa first if he needs it.

Pat: I think so, too.

Terese: Me, too!

Rosalie: What do you think, Mike? Mart?

Mike: You can just keep him here and you won't have to worry about it.

Rosalie: That's not the question. Of course we'll keep him here as long as we can. But I could never lift him. If it came to that . . .

Mart: How much is the house worth?

Milt: Wasn't it estimated at thirty-five to forty thousand, Marian? At two grand a month, that wouldn't last very long. He could live for a long time.

Mart: I think it's good that you're keeping him here, but the money is his as far as I'm concerned.

Terese: Nursing homes don't get enough money from people on public aid. That's why they don't have enough staff to take care of them. Don't ever put Grandpa into the Pinewood. That's a crummy place!

Rosalie: I think the proper thing to do would be to sell the house and put the money in his name in case we need it for him.

Milt: No, I don't want to do that. He has his pension and social security. That will pay part of it. I don't see why the house should be involved. As a son I am not liable for him, legally. He and Ma always said that house would be for you kids. That's the way it should be.

(*A brief silence*)

Cindy: How about if we play Uno?

Rosalie: That's a good idea. Who wants to play? Get it out, Cindy, and we'll see . . . .

So each time we arrived back at the same conclusion: we would keep Grandpa at home as long as possible, perhaps until some crisis came up that we could not handle ourselves. Meanwhile I placed his name on the waiting list at the county home, just in case.

A difference of opinion between Milt and myself always resulted in a delay, a postponement of decision making, because each of us was so concerned about our relationship that we didn't want to jeopardize it. So we continued to cope with each day's stresses as best we could, avoiding any real look toward the future.

Frequently, when Milt and I spoke with our friends about our situation, we joked about having a "two-year-old" again. In many ways Grandpa was like a child. He had to be helped to dress himself and to eat, and had to be told what he could touch and not touch. Like a two-year-old, Grandpa exasperated us and tried our patience continually with his rebellions and tantrums. In his case, however, the dependency gradually increased as time went on, shifting the balance between what he could do for himself and what we needed to do for him. It was important to me that he maintain as much independence as possible, but his confusion had increased so much that he seemed to be in a constant state of uncertainty. I resisted the impulse to button his clothes, tie his shoes, and so on, fearing that I might be the cause of his dependency, or that I might increase it. But I wanted to keep him calm and comfortable. Anything that made his life simpler simplified ours as well.

I had to watch my "two-year-old" pretty carefully, especially when he was quiet.

In one incident, Grandpa had wandered into the kitchen and was there alone for a few minutes when I realized I had better check on him. There he was, struggling to get a large roll of papers into his trousers pocket. My eyes moved to the table in front of him where the telephone book lay, open. Some fifty pages had been torn out.

Forgetting to be diplomatic, I grabbed for the roll of papers in Grandpa's hand. He resisted my grasp, and we played tug-of-war for a moment, while Grandpa found his voice: "You steal everything! That's mine! I need it! Bastar', you're no good! You steal!" The tirade went on and on while I went back to working at my desk in the family room. I could hear Grandpa fussing and fuming. The next thing I knew, he was going out the front door. After a minute I grabbed a jacket and followed after him. He was already across the street and heading toward the end of the block. He would not go back, no matter what I said to him. He was "going home." I would have to let him walk until he became tired, then get him back somehow.

I still didn't have an identification bracelet for Grandpa, and I never did get one. One reason was that he never went very far away, as some Alzheimer's patients do—boarding trains and busses and getting lost far from home. Another reason was that he would probably break it somehow and lose it. The police had been called to our aid several times—I was sure that they were aware of Grandpa's circumstances. If necessary, they would help us again.

Grandpa continued to "take off" frequently. Even that got to be routine! We were still giving him a tranquilizer pill every morning, but I often thought that it must be a very mild prescription because it didn't seem to have any effect. One day I made a comment about this to my friend Mary, and she corrected me. "That's a very powerful drug. It probably just isn't effective in Grandpa's case," she said. In January, with that in mind, I spoke to Milt, and we decided to try not giving Grandpa the tranquilizer pills for one month to see what would happen.

There was absolutely no visible change in Grandpa. We had stopped giving him the tranquilizer altogether. He was on no medication of any kind. At this point, we probably should have gone back to the internist with this information, but we did not.

During this period, Terese's early discovery that Grandpa liked to sing provided countless hours of enjoyment for him. Singing was something he could do for the family, a contribution he could make—a sense of usefulness was still important to him—and it helped him to pass the time as well. Sometimes he started singing on his own. Often one of us would ask him to sing. He would sing the same melody over and over, but no one seemed to mind. He was happy while he sang.

The photo album that had been a stimulant for early memories was now broken and torn, the pictures no longer meaningful to Grandpa. Now he was likely to tear off a corner of a picture and try to use it as a match to light his pipe. When he began tearing the pictures, I took the album away. It wouldn't be long before his special book would go the same way. Before that happened, Milt took the book to his office and made a photocopy of each page. He gave Grandpa the copy and filed the original away for posterity. Grandpa could still follow the words of the book to a limited extent, if someone helped him, but the book had lost most of its meaning for him.

The balloon game had now become the most useful way of interacting with Grandpa. There was always a blown-up balloon on top of our refrigerator, and whenever anyone had a few moments, a game with Grandpa would be in progress.

Cindy and her friend Jennifer devised a contest of their balloon-tossing skill; the winner would be whoever could get Grandpa to return the balloon with his left hand instead of his right the greatest number of times. They kept score. Because of the bursitis in his left upper arm, it was painful for Grandpa to raise his left arm, yet the exercise helped the circulation. Although he wouldn't consciously move the arm, in the midst of a game he became so intent on hitting the balloon that he didn't notice the soreness. Eventually the symptoms of bursitis pain were gone, thanks (I believe) to this simple balloon-tossing game.

Another discomfort Grandpa experienced was soreness of his feet due to bunions and occasional corns on his toes. Throughout these three and a half years, I had been making periodic trips to Cicero, taking him to the podiatrist near his old home. Somehow, though, the visits often got postponed; we or the doctor would be on vacation, or I would simply neglect to make an appointment. Moreover, each time we saw this doctor, he seemed to want to do more for Grandpa than I thought was necessary. For instance, he talked about all the surgery he had performed on people of all ages. For Grandpa he prescribed foot exercises. Now, if I had been determined, I probably could have found some way to get Grandpa to do these simple exercises, but it just wasn't worth the effort to me. Then the doctor suggested we buy an exercycle for Grandpa. That was the last straw! I knew he didn't have the vaguest idea what I was dealing with. I decided to find a more conveniently located podiatrist who might be better. All I wanted was someone who would take care of Grandpa's bunions and calluses and trim his toenails. Over the next few months I tried one new podiatrist, but I didn't like the setup there, so I looked for another. Finally I found a young man who was excellent: kind to Grandpa, patient with his occasional reluctance to cooperate, and very supportive. I was pleased that we had made this change, and we continued with this periodic treatment for as long as Grandpa stayed with us.

In the early spring, Milt and I were again involved in a series of classes for our church, this time a premarriage course for engaged couples, held in our home. It required at least one evening per week of preparation for the two of us, and one evening each week for six weeks, a small group of couples met in our home.

I had been concerned that Grandpa might interrupt our sessions by refusing to go to bed, but he did so only once. Actually, we could see that it was good for these young people to observe that we were taking care of Milt's dad. The purpose of the program was to help them gain a realistic, firsthand view of the factors involved in a successful marriage. Milt and I both felt we had something valuable to share with them.

Grandpa still "helped" me with my job of mailing chairperson for RE:AL. We spent one or two days at the center every other month or so, and although Grandpa could no longer help us with our work, he was content to think he was helping if I gave him a few defective sheets to fold. The ladies would cheer him on when he sang and pay attention to him when he tried to say something. It was becoming more difficult to keep him occupied long enough for me to finish the sorting at the end. Grandpa's restlessness was a problem in the large church hall where we worked. There were many places where he might wander, and the bathroom was far down the hall. We managed, however, to keep him near us without mishap. Once or twice I had to take him home before I was ready.

One of the big problems we had at this time was with Grandpa's bathroom visits. He was still continent, but the bladder control was weakening. The difficulty was that, although he knew when he had to go to the bathroom, the urge would come so fast, and he moved so slowly, that by the time he got to the bathroom, his clothes were a little wet. Or else he would get to the toilet all right, but once there, his poor eyesight and worse aim would result in a puddle of urine on the floor. Our bathroom had some loose floor tiles, and the urine would get underneath. Each time Grandpa wet the floor, I had to make a bleach solution and wash the toilet and floor, remove the loose vinyl tiles, wash underneath them, and put them back again. Otherwise the smell was very bad.

At this time, whenever the bell on the bathroom door sounded, Milt or I would rush to get there in time to turn Grandpa around so that he would urinate sitting down. Although this was more convenient for us, it seemed to be highly frustrating for him. Often a fight would ensue, and he would refuse to go at all. Then, of course, the whole scenario would be repeated five or ten minutes later. This went on for over a year. Grandpa finally became more accustomed to sitting down to urinate.

Two luncheons were coming up that spring, one at RE:AL

and the other sponsored by the Council of Catholic Women from our local parish. I wanted to attend both. I felt very fortunate indeed to find that I could. With more and more frequency I was calling on the two women whose names I had gotten from the church. One of them, Ann, refused to charge for her time. She said it was the only way she had of "doing something extra." She and her husband had no children; she had quit working and now had few obligations. She wanted to be home to serve dinner for her husband and to be with him in the evening, but other than that her time was her own, and she was usually available.

The other woman, Jane, had grown children but was now divorced and living alone. She made her living by caring for the elderly. She had other families who called upon her regularly, but whenever she was available, she was glad to stay with Grandpa. It felt very good to be able to attend these daytime functions, knowing that Grandpa was in good hands.

One evening when Cindy and I were alone and Grandpa had gone to bed, we got to talking about the fact that spring was here and that it made us feel ambitious and invigorated. Cindy suggested that she would like to make some changes in her bedroom—move out some remnants of Terese's belongings. Then she pointed out some things in the family room that "bugged" her. From there we progressed to brainstorming about things we could do to improve the whole house. We had a lot of fun with this—"rearranging" the living room furniture (without actually moving anything), making measurements, and playing around with several ideas. One of the ideas was to move the piano from the family room to the living room.

The more I thought about moving the piano, the more the idea took hold in my mind. We had bought a new piano when Cindy was in eighth grade, her teacher having noted that Cindy's progress in technique would be facilitated by a better instrument than our little spinet. Our lovely new piano had been placed in our small family room, where desk, sewing machine, file cabinets, table with chairs, and sundry other items were crammed together. This was where Cindy had to practice, while Grandpa interrupted frequently, or took her books and misplaced them. In addition, the high volume of her playing sounded harsh and jarring in the small room.

Cindy had never complained, but I felt strongly that moving the piano to the living room was a splendid idea. We had found a perfect spot for it, one that would necessitate only one other change. I was really excited to see what a difference it would make in the appearance of the room and the sound of the music.

There was just one problem. Milt believed that pianos did not belong in living rooms! It was his belief that people who had lots of money bought pianos just for show and displayed them proudly in a living room that was seldom even used, let alone lived in. The piano was just a prestigious piece of furniture. To avoid that kind of pretentiousness, he had developed the theory that pianos do not belong in living rooms. Now, however, I was sure that I could convince him otherwise.

The next morning, which was a Saturday, I shared with Milt all the fun Cindy and I had had with our fantasy of redoing various things in her bedroom, the family room, and the living room. Nonchalantly, I mentioned moving the piano. I was unprepared for the brick wall that suddenly appeared as Milt stated, "Obviously, pianos do not belong in living rooms." The fact that I had grown up with a piano in my living room was dismissed as an irrelevant statistic. Milt acted cool toward me for several days, or so I perceived it.

The next Sunday, Milt and I did some brainstorming ourselves about changes we could make in the house that spring. We got a little carried away too—planning to put a skylight in the kitchen! This was great!

I didn't mention the piano again until a later date, at a time when Milt and I were alone. I asked him to explain his statement that "pianos don't belong in living rooms." I listened carefully as he talked about it being a matter of "good taste." As he was about to go on with his ideas for the family room, I stopped him. I began my own treatise on "pianos as a part of the family circle—wherever that happens to be."

Milt suggested that I should "reeducate" myself, because obviously I had the wrong idea.

I surprised myself by remaining very calm as I pointed out that perhaps he could reeducate himself in this matter.

I suggested a possible compromise: since Cindy was the person who used the piano, and since having the piano in the living room would most directly benefit her, we could relocate the piano temporarily, for the three years remaining until Cindy would graduate from high school.

Milt was not interested in trying this temporary arrangement.

The sparring went on. I pointed out that he was not honoring my feelings in the matter. He insisted that it was his feelings that were not being honored.

I pointed out that his feelings had been honored for fifteen years. That was "beside the point."

Milt suggested that since we were still at loggerheads, we should end the discussion. I agreed. The climate was cool.

Later I was leaving to go to the store, and I was tempted to leave without a good-bye kiss. Instead, I told him, "I feel angry and disappointed, but I'll give you a kiss anyway," and I gave him a peck on the cheek.

Then next morning, a Sunday, Milt left for church while Grandpa and I sat outside in the warm May sunshine. I got out my journal and began writing. When Milt came home, he gave me a quick kiss, and I continued writing. He didn't ask me what I was writing—he didn't have to.

As I wrote, I began to sort out my options. I had to admit that there were a number of ways in which I could get back at Milt if I wanted to. But was that what I wanted? What about my feelings? Must I suppress them? Could I forget all this without a twinge of resentment?

I concluded that if I really meant it when I said, "Love is a decision"—if I really meant it when I said, "Lord, I give my life to you; you lead, I will follow"—then I must renounce my feelings of resentment. Even so much as putting them into words would be giving them power over me. Moreover, my marriage was (and is) extremely important to me, and I knew how "little things" could erode a relationship.

Later that afternoon I went shopping. When I returned, Milt had gone to some school affair, leaving an envelope for me on the kitchen table. Inside was a note which said: "Dear Rosalie, You had your opportunity to write earlier today. Now it is my turn to write. I'll be brief. I value our relationship more than the location of the piano. I love you. Milt."

When Milt came home, I greeted him with a kiss as always and told him that our relationship was important to me, too. Both of us, however, were distant for the rest of the day. When we went to bed, I reached as usual to hold his hand. We were quiet for a while, but gradually we began to talk. I told Milt that I was willing to forget the whole incident, but that I could not promise to forget it immediately—it would take time.

He was not expecting that kind of a response from me. I guess he thought that since he had given in, we would move the piano, and that would be the end of it. Instead, he felt that I was resentful and was trying to make him feel guilty. He couldn't handle that.

I tried to explain to him that, for me, the issue was more than just the location of a piece of furniture. It was that I had some very strong feelings about the matter, and he had dismissed them as unimportant. He hadn't even considered the compromise I offered; he had behaved as though his point of view was the only right one. This had been frustrating for me.

He still couldn't understand.

Then I drew a parallel, reminding him about his recent suggestion that I join him on a backpacking trip that summer, since he hadn't found anyone else to go with him. My first impulse had been to say, "No way!" Instead of saying it, however, I had let him explain what he had in mind. I had tried to listen not only to his words but also to his feelings. I had actually agreed to try backpacking again, in spite of a certain reluctance and even fear on my part.

Suddenly, he grasped what I was trying to say. He understood my frustration. Then he asked me to forgive him.

In a moment, tears gushed from my eyes and all my hurt feelings were washed away. We embraced and stayed in each others' arms, feeling really close, for some time. It was beautiful.

The concluding statement in my journal reads: "The reason we have been so successful in our relationship is that we both want so much to love and be loved by one another."

8 · The Fifth Year

I waken suddenly and glance at the clock: 5:05 A.M. I hear Grandpa's deep voice from downstairs saying, "I don't know where to go. . . . What can I do? . . . Where can I go? My, my. . . ." I lie there for a moment, mentally following him as he shuffles in stockinged feet, undershirt, and boxer shorts, bent figure leaning from the hips, hands groping for walls and furniture as he moves by inches from the bedroom, through the hall, toward the small glow of the night-light beside the bathroom door.

The voice becomes more insistent. "Where can I go? . . . Please? . . . Anybody there? . . ." I rise quickly now and, not bothering to put a robe over my nightgown, I go down the stairs and meet him in the hallway. Beckoning to him with my finger, I say only, "This way, Grandpa," and stand in front of the bathroom door, waiting. When he gets close enough, I point to the toilet and hope that he will know what to do there. If he doesn't, I help him to lower his shorts and sit down. Then I withdraw, sit on the stairs, and listen.

He continues talking. "I don't know what to do. . . . I don't know what to do. . . . My, my." I listen not only for his words but for the sounds of his bodily functions, which miraculously happen in spite of his confusion. Then I know that he will probably go back to sleep, and that I, too, can go back to sleep.

By the fifth year of his stay with us, Grandpa had become much more confused and withdrawn from what went on around him. Now Milt and I and the family seemed to be living from day to day a sort of humdrum acceptance, not too surprised about anything Grandpa did, resigned to the task of making his days as comfortable as possible, saddened by the inevitability of his continuing mental and physical deterioration.

Milt and I pursued our various interests, relegating to Grandpa only partially the hours we spent with him—we were half in attendance, half elsewhere, as it were. He was in his own world, we in ours; and if they didn't have to mix, so much the better.

As summer began, Terese went on a camping and canoeing trip to Missouri with a group from the university. She came home briefly and then left for Michigan, where she would work as a summer-camp counselor, something she had wanted to do since her early teens.

Mart, meanwhile, returned to a similar job in Wisconsin; Mike to the "Y" day camp in Elmhurst, still living at home. Although these jobs paid low wages and at times were very demanding, they at least provided a change of scene and an opportunity to be in the summer sunshine, working with other young adults and helping young children to enjoy the outdoors.

Up to this time, Grandpa had been no problem at night. Once he fell asleep, he would sleep soundly until about five o'clock, when he would get up and require some attention. Now, however, this pattern began to change. He began waking up at three or so, and instead of going back to sleep, he would lie in bed and talk, obviously unable to sleep. "My, my. . . . What shall I do? . . . My, my, what shall I do?" He went on and on. It was very annoying because it kept me awake, wondering what was the matter, whether he was getting out of bed, and if he somehow had to go to the bathroom again. Usually I would listen for a while and then go downstairs, take him to the bathroom, and put him back to bed, hoping that would end it. After a few minutes he'd start up again, like a radio that refused to be shut off. Two or three hours would go by before he fell asleep again, and by then it was time for me to be up for the day.

I was usually the one who tended to him when he woke up. If it was a particularly bad night, Milt would take his turn going downstairs too. I was reminded of the times, when our children were small, that Milt had boasted jokingly that he had a callus on his elbow from poking me in the middle of the night when the children needed attention. Now we were caring for his own father, and he still expected me to get up at night with him as well as take care of him during the day. Of course, we had never talked about this.

One particularly troublesome night, I had gone down to Grandpa three times and had gone back to sleep. I woke suddenly and heard him again. Sighing, I lay there, waiting to see whether Grandpa would stop or whether Milt would wake up and tend to him.

Finally, I got out of bed just as Milt also crawled out from the other side. Milt said to me sleepily, "I heard him, but I was down with him several times already, and I thought I'd just let him talk."

In surprise, I said, "Oh, I didn't know you were down with him already. I was down three times myself. I was waiting for you to wake up!"

Somehow that conversation in the early morning darkness shed new light on Milt's way of thinking. From that time on, he volunteered to do "night duty" with Grandpa and was also more attentive at other times when he was home.

This change in Milt's behavior meant a great deal to me. I could see that he really wanted to do his part in taking care of his father. We became closer as a result.

We had stopped giving Grandpa the tranquilizer medication in January because it didn't have any effect on his sudden spells of anger and his leaving home. As his nighttime wakefulness continued, Milt became more determined to prevent it somehow. He had listened to enough television commercials to be convinced that there must be some prescription drug or perhaps even an over-the-counter remedy for this.

In July I had a regularly scheduled appointment for Grandpa with Dr. Novak, the urologist. Something came up and I was unable to take Grandpa, so Milt did. He came home with a prescription for a popular tranquilizing drug. Milt had shared with Dr. Novak our difficulty with Grandpa's waking up at night, and the fact that at this point Grandpa was not under any particular doctor's care. He had requested a prescription for something that might help Grandpa to sleep.

First we tried one pill, but there was no change. The next

night we gave him two pills. Grandpa became very groggy, walked in a zig-zag, and before we had all gone to bed for the night, he had urinated all over the family-room floor. Clearly this was not the answer to our needs!

The problem was simply put on hold for a while, because it was time for Milt and two of his fellow educators and nature lovers to leave for Wyoming and some real mountain backpacking. One of the three had backpacking experience and willingly shared his expertise with the two neophytes. There were stories circulating about campers being mauled by bears, which led to some apprehension; but the only wild animals they actually encountered were in the Mangy Moose Saloon after the trail's end.

Shortly after Milt returned, he and I, together with Cindy and her friend Jennifer, drove to Washington, D.C., and Williamsburg, Virginia, for a nine-day family vacation. My friend Mary cared for Grandpa during the day, Monday through Friday, while Mike again did his part in the evenings and at night, with help from Marian and Pat on the two weekends.

For Milt, this trip was a double step back in time. A one-time history major, he doted on visiting any area of historic significance. Moreover, Washington and Williamsburg had been the sites of an annual eighth-grade class trip during his fifteen years as principal in his previous job. Far from being bored with going back again, he anticipated playing tour guide *par excellence*. His enthusiasm more than made up for Cindy's lack of it. We extended the invitation to Cindy's friend Jennifer in an attempt to make the trip more palatable for her. During the twenty-hour non-air-conditioned drive in 90-degree heat which began and ended our journey, the two girls sprawled in the back seat, their long legs and arms stretched out in all directions as they played games, read, or slept to pass the time. Once we hit the motel they emerged to banter, compete, and challenge one another with games and teasing, making good company with few complaints. Our country's capitol welcomed us, brilliant and vibrant both in sunshine and rain, as our personal tour guide led us to see the Senate and House chambers, White House, Lincoln and Jefferson memorials, and other places of interest. In Williamsburg we were fascinated by the reconstruction of a simpler life and life-style. An evening performance of ballads of the 1800s, performed by madrigal singers and accompanied by flutes, fifes, and early stringed instruments, carried us all on waves of harmony.

Cindy and Jennifer purchased fifes as souvenirs and entertained us thereafter with their determined efforts to produce chromatic scales and melodies.

During August of that year, I again attended the Christian Writers' Conference in Green Lake, Wisconsin. This time I chose a class in article writing instead of poetry. My topic was "Caring for an Aged Parent." I finished the article and later that month submitted it to a magazine for Christian families suggested to me as a possible market by my friend Mary. I was elated when it was accepted for publication.

Mid-August meant back to school for Milt; it was always a busy time of gathering materials, welcoming new teachers and families, and arranging for a smooth adjustment to a new year. Cindy returned to high school, Terese to Western Illinois University, Mike to his bus-driving job, and Mart, still not ready to return to school, to his simple life in Green Bay, Wisconsin. Marian and Jim celebrated their first wedding anniversary in June. Pat and John announced the happy news that they were expecting a baby in April. It would be our first grandchild—life continuing its cycle of renewal.

RE:AL followed the schedule of the school year, and as we began making plans for the fall brochure-mailing project, I realized I could no longer continue as chairperson of the mailing committee. It was becoming too frustrating for me to take Grandpa with me when I had to work at the Center. Sometimes he refused to go when I was ready, and people would have to wait for me; he was restless while he was there, and he was impatient to leave. I couldn't concentrate on the work. So I resigned from my responsibilities but continued to help the group until we could find someone else to take charge. The organization itself was experiencing difficulties, and I felt I could not give the amount of time that was required of me. I wrote my last newsletter for RE:AL later that fall.

As a result of our fantasies of the previous spring regarding our house, the piano now added a lovely new look and sound to the living room, and we had hired a contractor to make some exciting changes: a skylight to brighten our kitchen and a new rear doorway from the family room, which involved closing up the old entrance on the side of the house. How would Grandpa react to all of this? we wondered, hoping that it would not upset him too much.

The contractor delayed until November, and we were filled with misgivings about Grandpa's reaction to the disruption of routine and the intrusion of cold weather. Once the work was begun, however, the skylight was soon in place and the kitchen back to normal. The work in the family room took longer. Grandpa's response to the ladders, the noise, the men walking in and out, the plastic sheets tacked up to minimize the winter breezes in the house, was only, "What are they doing? . . . My, my." We were amazed that he was able to accept all of this going on without feeling threatened. It was evidence of the progression of his disease.

By this time we had long been convinced that Grandpa had Alzheimer's disease, although this had not been diagnosed by a doctor. Milt and I had been attending support group meetings of the ADRDA (Alzheimer's Disease and Related Disorders Association) for some time. Through this group, we had come to know about a neurologist who was particularly interested in Alzheimer's disease and who worked with several of the families represented in the group. Although this doctor's office was at some distance from us, I made an appointment to have him examine Grandpa. We met with Dr. James (a fictitious name) and explained the problems we had been having with Milt's dad both in the evening and during the night.

After Dr. James questioned Milt and me at length while Grandpa waited patiently in the next room, the three of us sat together once again while the doctor examined Grandpa, first physically and then with questions.

"Do you know your name?"

"Yes, sure."

"What is your name?"

Grandpa took some time before answering, while the question was repeated several times. Then, "Frank. Frank Honel."

"How old are you?"

"Eighty? . . . Ninety? . . . My, my." He was actually eighty-six.

"Who is this?" The doctor indicated Milt.

"My, my." Again, the question was repeated. "He's a good man."

"What is his name?"

"That's Milt. My, my."

Questions to bring out the relationship between Milt and Grandpa he could not answer, nor did he remember my name or our relationship. He did not know what day it was, or any information about current events. It was obvious that Grandpa had lost touch with what was going on in the world around him.

The doctor prescribed some specific blood tests that would rule out certain other factors, but on the basis of his consultation with us and his examination of Grandpa, he concluded that Grandpa did have senile dementia of the Alzheimer type.

Because of Grandpa's confusion and possible resistance, Dr. James noted that a full battery of neurological tests involving hospitalization was inadvisable and unnecessary. The diagnosis confirmed what we had long believed. Parts of Grandpa's brain were being destroyed by some strange accumulation of "plaques" and "tangles."* His attempts to deal with his surroundings in the face of this brain disfunction could explain many of the difficulties he experienced.

Dr. James suggested that we continue to experiment with various amounts of the drug we had purchased through Dr. Novak, giving it to Grandpa at bedtime and recording the results for eleven days. We did this and concluded at the end of that time that Grandpa's behavior had not changed significantly. He was still unpredictable, still refused to go to bed, still kept us awake with his loud talking at night. Moreover, there was one negative effect: his bladder control was definitely lessened. He couldn't make it to the bathroom without wetting himself, requiring numerous changes of clothing. We did not want that; so

*Mace and Rabins, The 36-Hour Day, p. 223.

we quit using the prescription, but somehow I put off calling Dr. James to report back to him.

Grandpa was always unpredictable, the friction between his will and ours unceasing. If we wanted to go somewhere and needed to take him with us, he refused to go. If I was in the middle of baking a cake, he got angry about something and stalked off down the street so that I had to chase after him. If he was quiet for a while and I was able to work on some project of my own—then I'd discover he had hidden some clothes or utensils, or some other valuables. If he picked up a magazine, he might roll it and stuff it into his pocket or tear some pages out. If I grabbed something out of his hands, as I often did, he'd shout and harangue at me, or we'd have a tugging contest over it. If we had company over for dinner, the meal could be interrupted by a big argument, making everyone tense and uneasy. Sometimes, when we held an evening meeting at our home, he picked that night to stage a strike against going to bed, and his loud voice and sporadic rambling phrases made it difficult for participants to hear each other and to concentrate on the subject of discussion—not to mention that Milt or I would have to jump up every few minutes to tend to him. There were times when we got so tired of dealing with him by nighttime that we turned out all the lights downstairs and hid ourselves in our bedrooms so he'd think we had gone to bed! (This didn't work either, because I had to creep downstairs every few minutes to see what this ungainly hulk was doing, rambling around in the dark. I wasn't even worried that he would fall or hurt himself.) The strain of having this strong, uncontrollable "child" challenged Milt and me and every person in our family constantly.

That fall the ADRDA organized a publicity campaign to bring Alzheimer's disease to the attention of the public. Members were encouraged to try in all possible ways to publicize the need for research into the causes and treatment of Alzheimer's disease and the plight of families caring for its victims. The month of November was chosen as a time for a coordinated effort. I felt that I had been helped a great deal by ADRDA and by the newspaper publicity that had originally brought it to my attention. My involvement in the support group and in various informative meetings held for all of the Chicago area had helped me and my family to learn more about the disease and methods of coping with the problems it caused. In order to do my part in the publicity effort, I telephoned our local newspaper and suggested they run an article on the disease during November. When asked why the issue was important to me, I answered that I was caring for an Alzheimer's patient in my home. Would I be willing to be named and photographed? I said that I would. A reporter was assigned to do the story. I supplied her with factual information about the numbers of people affected, symptoms and difficulties, community resources available, and the need for further efforts on behalf of patients and their families. A picture of Grandpa and me playing the balloon-toss game was used with the article.

As a result of the publication of that article, Milt and I received responses from a number of people who wanted more information about contacting the ADRDA and support groups in our area. People not only asked us questions but also shared their stories with us and began sending us articles on Alzheimer's disease from all sorts of publications.

During the Christmas season, beginning in mid-December, Grandpa's sleep pattern again changed radically. Probably because he wasn't sleeping well at night, he would be exhausted by dinner time, five or six o'clock, so he would go to bed right after dinner. Then about an hour later he would wake up and be ready to be entertained. He wandered about looking for us, either wanting something to do or demanding to "go home." Many times he went out into the night, sometimes in his stockinged feet, even when the weather was severely cold or when ice and snow were on the ground. (His shoes were off because he had been in bed for the night.) Milt let him go outside like that, figuring that Grandpa would get cold and come back in right away. Mike voiced loud complaints at that treatment, and I agreed with him, but when Milt was handling Grandpa, he tolerated no interference. Grandpa never suffered any harm from these brief sorties into the night.

I well remember one night when I was really exasperated with him. I was wearing a new pair of flannel pajamas, perhaps for the first time. Their purchase had represented a deliberate choice of comfortable, rather than attractive, nightclothes for myself, for I was learning to be more conscious of my own needs and more assertive in looking after them.

That day, Grandpa had had a quiet morning followed by an afternoon of anxiety and hyperactivity. I took him shopping, hoping to wear him out, and he picked some things off the shelves in the store, something he had never done before. He said he was hungry, so I selected a box of cookies, opened the box, gave him several cookies, and continued with my shopping. When we got to the frozen-food counter, he grabbed a box of vegetables and wouldn't let me put it back. He held it in one hand, pushing the cart awkwardly with the other. At that point, I realized that this trip was not going to work, so I steered him to the checkout counter while he clung to the box. He refused to give it to the cashier or to allow either of us to see what it was so that she could charge me for it. (She finally did.) This cashier and all the store's employees were familiar with us because we shopped there so often. They were very patient and understanding, but I felt tense and anxious because of the disturbance. We got back in the car and drove home, Grandpa still holding onto his now-thawing frozen vegetables. It was one of the few times I had not been able to complete my shopping mission.

At dinner time, Grandpa was falling asleep. He would eat a bite or two of food, then his eyes would droop and his chin drop, and he would sit silently, dozing. Milt and I kept talking to him to rouse him. As soon as we had finished eating, I took him to the bathroom and then to bed. He went to sleep immediately.

It was still early in the evening when I heard Grandpa's voice. Soon he was up. I took him to the bathroom and led him back to bed again. He was wide awake and had no intention of going to sleep. "Okay, Grandpa, you don't have to go to bed if you don't want to," I said, but inwardly I was wishing that I could lock him in his room and make him stay there. I sat down at my desk in the family room to read, so I would be near him.

"I ain't got nothing. Nothing to eat," he said, sitting at the table with his piles of paper.

I fixed him some bread and jelly.

"You eat, too," he said, "Here." He held up a bite on his spoon for me.

"No thanks, Grandpa. I ate already."

He got up to bring me a bit of his bread. I knew he wouldn't leave me alone, so I went into the kitchen. Soon he finished eating and came into the kitchen also. We played balloon-toss for a while. Then I tried taking him to bed again, but he wouldn't stay.

When Milt came home from his Parent-Teacher Association meeting at ten o'clock, Grandpa was still bright-eyed and anything but sleepy. We sat and visited for a while, had a cup of hot chocolate together, and tried again. Grandpa seemed to be quiet, so we went upstairs to get ready for bed ourselves.

I was just falling asleep when I heard him again, saying, "My, my, . . . What shall I do?"

Startled awake, I sighed as the realization hit me. "Oh, no, not again!" I muttered. Reluctantly, I went downstairs—in my new pajamas—to find him already in the hall.

"Grandpa, it's time to go to sleep!" I said sternly. "Now go back to bed!" He tried to go past me, so I took him determinedly by the two arms and turned him around, heading back to his bedroom. "Now sit here on the bed, and I'll bring you something good," I told him. I got a juice glass from the kitchen, went downstairs to the bar, and put a little sweet wine into the glass. Then I handed it to him. He took a gulp, winced, and choked a little.

"Strong!" he said, and drank some more. He finished the wine. I took the glass from him. He started to stand up.

"No!" I said. "You go to sleep now, you hear?" I felt anger boiling up in me as he tried to get up again. I struggled to make him lie down, pushing him with all of my strength. Somehow his foot caught in the leg of my pajamas, and in the scuffle the new fabric tore a jagged two inches up from the bottom. I won the battle. Grandpa was lying down on his bed, breathing hard.

"Now stay there!" I said, and glared at him. Then I turned out the light and closed the door.

My energy was spent. I felt chagrin as I examined the extent of damage to my pajama leg. "Why was I so angry?" I asked myself. "I'm lucky he didn't hit his head on the bed." I could envision him lying there in a pool of blood, and I prayed for mercy and forgiveness.

I went back upstairs and tried to sleep. It was no use. Sure enough, there he was again: "My, my. . . . What shall I do?"

"Well, Lord, I guess you're giving me another chance," I smiled to myself. I decided to wait a while before going back down again.

Milt stirred and said, "Let's leave him alone for a while; then I'll go down."

"Thanks," I said.

Years later I still wear that pair of pajamas, and it serves as a reminder to me of my many failures—of how easy it is to succumb to cruelty and impatience, to selfishness, rather than to respond with unconditional love.

Scenes like this one didn't happen every night. Perhaps five out of ten nights, Grandpa went to bed at seven and slept, leaving us free to enjoy a peaceful evening. Milt and I, however, obstinately resisted accepting the 50 percent chance of having a free evening. In the event there was someplace we both wanted to go, and I didn't have, or couldn't find, a sitter, we had to decide in advance which one of us (usually Milt) would stay home. When we were both at home and Grandpa stayed up late, we would often withdraw to a remote part of the house to watch television, checking on him at intervals. Poor Grandpa! As Mike said later, we "consistently ignored and mistreated him."

A brief note in my journal at that time read:

Grandpa's evening and nighttime sleep habits periodically challenge us and try our patience to the utmost. I often wish for a soundproof, padded cell that I could lock him in! How Milt and I long for a whole night of uninterrupted sleep! As parents of six children, being awakened and kept up at night is not new to us, but we look forward to the time when this burden will pass, when our life will return to "normal" again; when our days will be freed of the constant friction and tension that stem from having Grandpa in our home.

On Christmas Eve Milt and I were home alone with Grandpa. He went to bed nicely. That afternoon, Terese and Mart had left for the "sibling party" at Pat and John's. Cindy had to sing in the folk choir at the 5:15 Mass, so she and Mike drove to the party afterward. They brought sleeping bags and pillows. Marian and Jim had invited Milt and me to attend Midnight Mass with them in Cicero after they returned from Jim's family's Christmas Eve party. We went, leaving Grandpa asleep and the doors bolted. When we all got together the next day, someone asked, "Are we going to the nursing home again?"

The response was mixed and not very enthusiastic. It was as if we were compelled to repeat an unpleasant obligation.

"We don't have to go."

"No, but I think we should."

"I'm not so sure I want to go there this year."

"We didn't make any gifts to bring."

"That's okay, we can still go."

"Let's take a vote." The majority voted in favor of going. I abstained.

"We didn't call to ask if we could go."

"I'll call." Milt went to the phone. It was all right for us to go. Grandpa refused at first to put on his coat and walk to the car, but with some effort, I was able to persuade him. When we got to the nursing home, he was reluctant to move, walking very slowly, stopping frequently. Since he was considerably weaker than a year ago, someone suggested that he sit in a wheelchair so that he could keep up with us as we walked down the hallways singing our carols. Grandpa didn't like it. He kept getting up and urging someone else to sit in the chair so he could push them. One of the patients joined us and pushed another wheelchair patient along in our procession. With all of this, we made slow progress, so after twenty or twenty-five minutes we decided to leave. It seemed to me in retrospect that Grandpa may have reacted as he did because he didn't want to be considered helpless. Maybe he was afraid we would leave him at the nursing home. At any rate, we should have let him walk. He was not ready for a wheelchair.

After the holidays, Milt and I were still in disagreement concerning what we should do about Grandpa's change of sleep habits. Milt wanted me to call Dr. James for a different medication, while I delayed, feeling that medication was not the answer for us. I was discouraged by the failure of our previous attempts to change Grandpa's behavior through medication. Moreover, it was my personal philosophy not to depend on drugs if at all possible.

The difficulty in medicating for Alzheimer's disease stems from the fact that so little is known about the cause of the disease; there is no treatment for the disease itself. The most common use of drugs in cases of Alzheimer's disease is in the management of behavior problems such as psychological depression, agitation, sleeplessness, and paranoia, which are treatable with psychoactive drugs, often, unfortunately, with undesirable side effects.*

There is no easy answer to these problems, since the brain chemistry and bodily reaction of every individual is different. Regardless of whether medication is used, it is still necessary for the caretakers of an Alzheimer's patient to cope and manage and respond in various ways to various situations to achieve the desired results: manageable behavior.

Finally, in late January, I called Dr. James again. He prescribed a tranquilizing drug that was different from either of the two we had tried previously, which had been ineffective. This time there seemed to be some improvement. Grandpa's sleepless nights were less frequent. We tested different dosages of the tranquilizer, according to Dr. James' instructions. There were no apparent side effects. We continued using this medication daily.

It was seven o'clock in the evening, Grandpa's bedtime. I took him by the hand and asked him to come with me. He complied, shuffling slowly around table and chairs, down the three steps leading from the kitchen. I took him to the bathroom and sat him on the toilet, but nothing happened. After a brief wait I got him up, dressed him, and took him to his bedroom. He needed some help removing his shoes. I assured him that I would "save them" for him till the morning. I gave him his pill embedded in a bite

*Robert D. Terry, M.D., and Robert Katzman, M.D., "Senile Dementia of the Alzheimer Type," *Annals of Neurology*, Nov. 1983, p. 502.

of banana. As he chewed the banana I lifted his legs onto the bed, causing him to lower his head, though reluctantly, to the pillow.

After putting the light out, I returned to his bedside and took his hand in mine while stroking his shoulder gently and saying, "Good-night, good-night." I could tell he was agitated, however, because he grabbed at my hand and arm with stiff, jerky movements and didn't want to let go.

For what seemed a long while I stood there, allowing him to fondle my hand and arm, waiting for him to calm down. He didn't.

Then I left, and I could hear him talking after the door was closed. "My, my. My, my, What is it? I can't. I can't. I have to get up. I have to get up. . . ."

Sure enough, after a minute he was back in the hall. I had to leave for a meeting, so Milt took him to the bathroom. When I returned from my meeting at nine o'clock, Grandpa was in the bathroom again, having spent the interim in and out of bed and bathroom, or just sitting with Milt. This time when Milt put him to bed again, he stayed for the night.

I felt very thankful for Milt's willingness to spend a greater amount of his time with Grandpa. Very often the two would sit at the kitchen table together, Milt holding Grandpa's hand as he read a book or magazine in the evening. There were fewer arguments between them.

Confrontations between Milt and Mike were now rare. My own relationship with Mike was strengthened by my appreciation that I had another person around to help entertain Grandpa. Mike had found many other outlets for his energy, but he looked for every opportunity to make Grandpa laugh, dressing him up in silly hats and scarves, taking his picture in different poses (which Grandpa loved), shaking hands in their special way. While Milt and I felt we had to raise our voices to make Grandpa understand us, Mike spoke close to his ear in a normal tone and he understood.

Communication had improved between my son and me also. Mike tended toward vegetarianism, and in order to have the kinds of meals he wanted, he got involved in cooking. He was what you might call an unorthodox cook. He read books on vegetarianism and nutrition and translated these into rice and bean dishes with spicy sauces that Milt and I gradually learned to relish, though at first we would only taste them. He and I came up with some meals that were a compromise between his far-out tendencies and my conservatism. When Mike convinced his dad to relinquish complete control of the vegetable garden in our backyard, we enjoyed the fruits of his efforts in a great variety of salads and vegetable dishes through summer and fall.

At age twenty-five, however, Mike had been pondering his future and was becoming restless about living at home. His interest in biology was still strong, and his work with schoolchildren as a bus driver was beginning to lead him toward teaching as a possible career. But he also had a desire to travel. Now he made plans to take a two-month camping trip alone by car. He headed south on February 1 in order to see the early-spring bird migrations as he pitched his tent in state-park campgrounds in southern Illinois, Arkansas, and Louisiana. His first main destination was Houston, Texas, where he stayed with my sister Pat for a few days before continuing south to Padre Island. There he visited some extraordinary bird sanctuaries and added many new sightings to his "life list." During his trip, he also visited family friends in Georgia, and my brother and his family in Ohio; and for one week he joined a volunteer work crew in Appalachia. When he telephoned, the first thing he always asked was "How's Grandpa?" He really missed his pal.

Meanwhile because of our membership in ADRDA, Grandpa, Milt, and I had been invited to participate in a segment of a Chicago television news show. We agreed, and on the scheduled day a television crew consisting of a woman reporter, a cameraman, and a sound technician came into our home with all of their equipment. The reporter met Grandpa, asked us some preliminary questions, and quickly refreshed her makeup. On camera, we were asked various questions about our experience with Grandpa and our reasons for taking care of him at home. Some of the questions were repeated while the camera focused on the reporter and again on one of us. Sometimes the camera focused on Grandpa. Later we were notified when the segment would be shown. It had been cut and edited, of course, and other people had been interviewed also. It made a very interesting eight-minute news feature. Again, we felt that our public exposure was a way of helping other people who had problems similar to our own.

Since Grandpa had started waking up periodically during the night, now he often slept later in the morning. One day I recorded the following in my journal:

> Grandpa woke up at about eight o'clock, talked a while ("What shall I do? Where shall I go? . . ."), and came out of his bedroom; I directed him to the bathroom. "This?" he asked, pointing to the toilet.
>
> "Open this up," I said, tapping his belt. He did, but didn't proceed to open pants and zipper. "More yet," I said, using his terminology. "Now drop the pants down." He did. "Now this"—underwear—"Now sit down."
>
> "How long?" he wanted to know. I didn't answer, because I had gone to another room. "How long shall I stay here?" he kept asking until I returned.
>
> I rephrased my answer several times before he could understand: "A little while. Until you are finished. I'll let you know." That satisfied him.
>
> Actually he sat there for two or three minutes, then got up, calling me: "What'll I do now? No shoes."
>
> I brought his shoes for him to put on, and then gave him a piece of bread with jelly and a glass of milk. He was quiet there for a while.
>
> Later I heard him go into the bathroom (the bell rang on the door), and I heard the swishing sound of water. He had "washed" his plate—and probably his cup also—in the toilet water. I took them from him, explaining, "We don't do that. Let me wash them." I didn't mean to let my irritation show, because I realized he didn't know any better. But he knew I didn't like it.
>
> "I don't understand. What's wrong?" he kept saying, over and over.

Grandpa had become increasingly dependent, his knowledge of the simplest procedures lost. He constantly amazed me, however, with how well he could read my feelings.

Grandpa's days were an endless stream of monotony from my viewpoint, but he seemed unaware of the tedium. He just sat looking out of the dining room window, remarking when he saw a car go by, or a person walking, wondering out loud whether the person was coming to visit us. Sometimes he would watch the yellow fire hydrant on the corner, thinking it was a young person. He wondered why that "boy" was standing there so long—perhaps he was waiting for someone. He would say this over and over, wanting me to come and look at the boy, becoming annoyed if I did not.

The Fire Hydrant

Look
Come and see
A boy is standing there, waiting
I could go
and find out . . .

For vacant hours through endless days he sits
with dimmed demented gaze, at the window
seeking . . . something . . . someone
from a past eradicated page by page.

It's cold
See the snow?
A boy is standing there, waiting
Maybe he is lost
Maybe he has no place to go . . .

Can't you see?
You don't care.
I'm going!
I'm going home
Someone is there, waiting . . .

Grandpa had now lost the ability to comprehend written words and pictures and his photographs. He occupied himself at length with bits of paper. He would fold them or tear them into smaller pieces and then arrange them (sometimes like a collage, sometimes in various piles), put them in his pocket, or use them to wrap a spoon or dish. I recalled the years before he became ill, when he was widowed and living alone. His dining room table had always been covered with neat stacks of mail, photos, coupons, papers he had been looking at or sorting through, and things he wanted to give to us when we visited. It intrigued me that he continued doing these things that had lost all meaning, doing them simply by rote.

This aspect of Grandpa was not as difficult to accept, though it was tedious and demanding and unceasing, as the side of him that was stubborn and irritable, totally unreasonable and irrational. The disease seemed to have magnified both sides of his personality to extremes.

It's hard to tell someone unfamiliar with Alzheimer's disease just what it is that makes caring for an Alzheimer's sufferer difficult. Grandpa didn't look sick. Physically he was in excellent condition for his age, and his health had actually improved in some ways because we had been able to control his diet. When we took him to the store or other public places, he was seen as a fairly normal elderly person. He shuffled along slowly, not lifting his feet, but when people spoke to him, he usually responded in a normal way. When he saw children in the store, he would stop to smile at them and say a word or two as any kindly grandpa might do. Now, however, he did have the peculiar habit of talking audibly and constantly as he pushed the shopping cart. One of my friends said to me, "I always know when you're in the store because I can hear Grandpa saying 'My, my,' as he goes along." In addition, he did occasionally become hostile and uncooperative in a public place, so that we had to leave abruptly.

There was another dimension to our grocery-shopping trips which I believe needs to be mentioned. People in the two grocery stores in the neighborhood became accustomed to seeing us there. The cashiers, the managers, and many of the shoppers responded at various times and in different ways. They spoke to Grandpa and affirmed him by paying attention to him. Moreover, his presence provided a reason for communicating with me. Many people told me their story of someone Grandpa reminded them of—a parent, a spouse, or some other relative whom they cared for, or who was now or had been in a nursing home. It made me realize what an ordinary thing this was that I was doing, yet extraordinary, too, as people said, "I know what you're going through. I know how hard it is." These people were total strangers to me, yet somehow Grandpa was a connecting link to something deep inside us all. I felt thankful that I could be a witness of Christian love to these strangers and others who saw us.

There were further signs of Grandpa's continuing decline: he could no longer use his dentures properly. He had worn an upper denture plate for many years, and gradually he had lost his lower teeth, too. He was in his early seventies when the last three or four had been removed, and at that time he decided he was too old "to get his money's worth" from a new denture plate. He managed to eat without a lower plate.

Each evening we asked Grandpa for his dentures, which he would place in the proffered cup to be cleaned and soaked until morning. Eventually his mental state got to the point where he would take the teeth out and hide them, sending me rummaging through his drawers; or he was reluctant to remove them for cleaning, and I had to plead with him or reach into his mouth to loosen them for him. Finally, it happened that for several days he refused to take his teeth out at all, nor would he let someone else take them out. They remained in his mouth until he developed a soreness in his gums. It was so painful that he finally let me take the teeth out. The gums healed, and after that I never gave the dentures back to him again. He simply had to eat softer food.

It was easy enough to soften his slice of whole-grain bread by putting a little milk on it, then the topping of jelly or applesauce or stew. He still ate with a spoon and managed to chew to some extent. He seemed perfectly content without any teeth.

Grandpa didn't care to smoke as much as he used to. In fact, he began hiding his pipe, so I put it away in a safe place for him. Then if he asked for it I got it out, lit it for him and put it away again when he'd finished. Sometimes he complained that it didn't taste good anymore.

An identification with the senior-citizen set had been creeping gradually into my consciousness. At about the time of my mother's death, I hit the age of forty, and I realized soon afterward that I needed glasses for reading. Rather than have to take them off and put them on all the time, I opted for bifocals. More than a decade later, both of my parents were gone, and I saw myself as definitely a part of the new "older" generation—though still clinging to "middle-aged" status.

I had been thinking about trying contact lenses sooner or later—and my advancing age seemed to indicate that sooner would be better. My glasses were such a bother, always sliding down my nose, and it was about five years since I'd had my eyes checked. One day, when I saw an ad for contact lenses at a very reasonable price offered by an optician in a shopping center several miles away, I picked up the phone on an impulse and made an appointment to check it out.

The day of the appointment was a cold February day. In spite of the cold, of course, I had to take Grandpa with me. I had a little difficulty locating the shopping center—drove past it and had to turn around and go back—since the area was unfamiliar to me.

The shopping center was enormous, and although it was mid-afternoon on a weekday, the parking lot was jammed with cars. I had to park quite some distance from the entrance. There was no bench in front of the entrance, and I was afraid to leave Grandpa standing alone, so I parked and he walked with me to the entrance. It was a long walk for him, without a grocery cart to lean on. When we got inside, I discovered that there were numerous stores around a mall, and we had another distance to walk. I was not sure where the optical store was, so I led Grandpa to a nearby bench, and he sat to rest while I located the place I wanted. Already I was regretting making an appointment in this out-of-the-way place.

Finally I located the store and went back for Grandpa. We walked to the store together and I seated him in a comfortable chair in the waiting area. He didn't want to take his coat off, so I simply unbuttoned it. Then I gave him my purse to hold for me, a usual procedure in a case like this. A year ago I would have given him his book to hold and to read, but now it was my purse. He felt he was helping me by holding it for me.

I submitted my name and was asked to wait, so I sat next to Grandpa and picked up some brochures that told me the benefits of several different kinds of contact lenses. Finally it was my turn, and I was taken into a back-room area for an eye exam, not included in the sale price, of course. I felt a little taken in by that but figured it was time for one anyway. After the exam, I had to decide what kind of contacts I wanted (no refunds or exchanges). That was difficult. I asked many questions. Then the optometrist allowed me some time to think while she examined someone else. After making my selection, I was sent back to the outer room to wait until someone could help me with the actual contact lenses. The waiting area was not filled, but there were several people there. Grandpa was sitting quietly, holding my purse. I asked him if he wanted to walk a little. He didn't.

The wait was much longer than I had anticipated. I kept looking at my watch, hoping Grandpa didn't have to go to the bathroom, and envisioning getting stuck in rush-hour traffic on our way home. Still we waited.

Finally I decided to give up the whole thing. I went to the desk and explained that since I had my father-in-law with me, I would have to leave and come back some other time. That was fine, but since I had already had the eye exam I was asked to pay for it now. Okay, no problem. My checkbook was in my purse.

"Grandpa, I need this a minute, okay?" I said to him.

"No!" he answered, clamping his hands even more firmly on my purse.

"Oh, boy, what do I do now?" I said to myself. I sat down beside him to think.

"Grandpa," I said in the sweetest tone of voice I could muster, "I need something from my purse. I won't take it from you. Please let me just open it."

"No! It's mine! You steal!" he shouted.

I looked around to see who had heard this declaration. There were several people who had obviously sized up the situation I was in. I caught some smiles of sympathy and returned them sheepishly.

I waited a minute or two, thinking that Grandpa might loosen his grip and I could make a grab for my purse. I waited some more. He sat like a stone Buddha, every once in a while uttering his usual "My, my," his two hands firmly gripping the purse.

I went to the desk, which was located out of sight of this drama, and explained that they would have to send me a bill for the exam. That was quite all right. Then I went back to Grandpa and told him that I was finished here, and we could go home now.

"No! I'll stay here."

"Grandpa, don't you understand? We can go home now! Come with me. Get up!"

"No! I'll stay here. You go yourself."

By now a bit of panic was setting in. I had been in some interesting situations with Grandpa before, but none quite like this.

"Okay, Grandpa, then I'm going. Goodbye." I was using the threat-of-abandonment tactic. I walked out of the doorway and around the corner of the glass partition. I watched to see what Grandpa would do.

He didn't even look up. I stayed there for a couple of minutes. Then I went back inside and tried again. No success.

Summoning up all my courage and strength, I pounced on my purse and pulled as hard as I could. Grandpa pulled, too, but finally I got the purse away from him and slung it over my shoulder. Then I yanked and tugged at him by his upper arms (through his coat) until he was standing stiffly in front of the chair.

"Come on, Grandpa, we're going home."

He wouldn't move. I pulled him forward so that he was off balance and had to take a step. Then I got behind him, grabbed both upper arms firmly, and proceeded to push and shove him along from behind. (I had learned this trick from Milt.)

We had a long way to go. I knew I could never get him all the way to the car like this, so I steered him to the benches inside the entrance, which seemed to be a block away. We finally made it. Grandpa sat heavily.

I raced to the car and pulled it up to the curb in front of the entrance, leaving my trouble lights flashing. Again Grandpa refused to move. He was in a sort of stupor. I yanked him to his feet and pushed him step by step to the doorway. Someone held the door for us, and I got him outside. The cold air seemed to revive him somewhat, and when I opened the car door for him, he got in.

I breathed a sigh of relief and realized, as I started driving again, that I was shaking.

The rush hour was in progress. We made our way slowly along the highway, stoplight after stoplight. I turned on the radio for some calming music for both of us. The long ride gave me a chance to reflect.

I had learned several things from this experience, not the least of which was to make sure I was familiar with the place we were going before taking Grandpa.

I also realized that I might be entitled to a handicapped permit, so I phoned the city the next day and was told that I would need a doctor's signature on an application. I picked up an application form shortly thereafter, called Dr. James, and explained the situation. He agreed to sign for me, and I was issued a permit that was good for one year. I kept it in the glove compartment of the car and used it only when I felt it was really necessary.

Later I went back to the optical store without Grandpa and purchased my bargain-price contacts. They were awful. I followed the directions and wore them for a few hours every day for a week or two, but I couldn't get used to them, and it seemed to take forever to get them in and out. Perhaps I wasn't very highly motivated, for I soon decided it wasn't such a chore to push my glasses up again when they slipped down my nose.

As spring approached, Milt once again began to talk excitedly about going backpacking. His two friends from last year's trip were eager to go out west again this summer, and there were others who had become interested, as Milt shared his enthusiasm at any and every social gathering. Milt was the acknowledged leader of the group; he set up planning meetings, called everyone by phone, and recorded the progress they made in their plans.

Also at this time, many of the Catholic churches in our area were beginning a three-year program of renewal, called RENEW, something I had been reading about with interest in our diocesan newspaper. I felt it would be very beneficial for people in our parish, and Milt agreed. The laity would be asked to provide leadership in many areas, so we attended some of the early promotional meetings. We were then asked to chair the committee for planning large group activities in our parish. The focus of the overall program would be in small groups, but large group activities would be used periodically to build momentum and integrate the program. Milt and I would also be members of one of the small groups. This involvement provided a new outlet for our time and energy, especially for mine. I was pleased that Milt was willing to participate with me and that we would be working together.

While this new involvement in church programming began for me, another period of my life came to a close with the disbandment of the RE:AL organization in the spring. It seemed that a whole new gamut of enrichment classes and opportunities for women had arisen in our community, and RE:AL, which had been one of the first organizations to offer programs of this type, could no longer attract enough participants to continue its activities. This was another step in the cycle of change. Typically, while this change had evolved around me, I had moved in new directions, as had most of the women I had worked with in RE:AL. It was with sadness that we saw the end of an organization that had played an important part in our lives, but at the same time we knew that we must continually relinquish the old and reach toward the new. Many of the things I had learned through RE:AL were still being put to use in a variety of ways.

Meanwhile, Mike returned from his travels. He spoke excitedly about his many experiences, about being treated royally by relatives and friends, and about solving or surviving problems with his car, the theft of his wallet, and his loneliness. His week as a volunteer in Appalachia had enriched his understanding of the complex problems of poverty, and he described what he had seen firsthand: joblessness, destitution, shockingly bad living conditions, and adults and children suffering mental retardation due to malnutrition. The bird-watching segment of his trip had been highly successful. Besides the migration of warblers and other small birds, he had seen flocks of pelicans, ibis, cranes, and many other exotic specimens, and he had exchanged stories with other experienced "birders."

On Easter we gathered as a family, but without Terese, who was having exams and couldn't come so far just for the two-day weekend, and Mart, who stopped by on Friday to borrow our small car so that he could drive to West Virginia for a friend's wedding. Marian and her husband Jim showed pictures of their recent vacation trip to San Francisco, while Mike told of his adventures camping and visiting in Texas and Ohio with the aunts and uncle we don't see very often. Grandpa ate with us and sat in the living room afterward as we talked together.

With us that evening were a young couple, longtime friends of our daughter Pat and son-in-law John, with their two little girls. One of the little girls, a two-year-old, was frightened at first by Grandpa's loud voice. Gradually her fear subsided, and she watched him from afar with her big brown eyes and serious expression. John had brought a video player, which he hooked up to our television so that we could all watch a videotape of our news feature interview on Alzheimer's disease, which our support-group leader had made for us.

Just a few days later our first grandson, Shawn, was born, a healthy and beautiful baby, a miracle and a blessing. We acknowledged this new life as a gift, praising and thanking God in our hearts. Pat remarked that she had gained a new appreciation for my role of mother—an appreciation which continued to grow through the adjustment to tiredness, lack of sleep, and constant demands that the new parents had to make. I felt renewed in spirit by the tremendous joy of holding that small child of my child in my arms. Milt, too, was deeply touched by this new experience, and many memories of our own babies were brought to mind.

Cindy's sixteenth birthday fell on Mother's Day, and Shawn was one month old, making for a manifold celebration of family life. Grandpa posed with Milt, Pat, and Shawn for a four-generation picture. It also marked another step in the cycle of change: the end of Grandpa's fifth year with us.

9 ▪ The Sixth Year

It is a quiet evening. Grandpa went to bed on time, at seven o'clock. Putting him to bed has been difficult since a week ago Saturday, when daylight saving time began. Now I have newspaper taped to his bedroom window. Otherwise there would be too much light in there on a sunny evening like this one, even with the drapes closed.

Grandpa has slowed down perceptibly. He just sits doing nothing for a lot more of the time. However, he can still push the grocery cart up and down the aisles, and he doesn't complain.

Yesterday I had several errands other than grocery shopping to do, and I left him in the car for most of them. When we got to the post office, however, I brought him inside with me for some exercise. He got tired standing in line with me (the stamp and parcel windows were busier than usual), so he wandered into the other section. When I was finished I went to get him, but he refused to leave. Several people who had been in line with me also had business there, and they nodded to me or smiled in recognition. I waited in the vestibule for a few minutes, then went back and tried again, with the same result. He just stood there. The third time, he started to follow me until he saw that the pavement outside was wet from an earlier rain shower. He refused again. This time I pulled him forcefully forward and out the door. Then he began to cooperate. Someone who had observed all this remarked to me something about having a lot of patience. I am not sure I was being patient. I don't know what other recourse I had.

Another year had begun, another summer. Our daughter Pat and her husband, John, invited all of our family and all of John's family to celebrate Shawn's christening. John has four sisters and one brother, all married and with children. His family is a close-knit one; they relish get-togethers and provide many opportunities for the cousins—eleven in all now—to know each other well. John's parents are challenging role models for Milt and me in our new career as grandparents.

The christening itself took place in early afternoon, with the proud parents and grandparents and most of John's and Pat's siblings present. John's youngest sister and our son Mike served as godparents. Baby Shawn was dressed in a christening dress that had previously been worn by forty-five babies in John's family, reaching back two generations. The party that followed was a lovely large-family affair with gifts and food brought by everyone, and children roaming everywhere in high excitement. It was wonderful, and I was thankful that I had been able to find a sitter to stay with Grandpa. It would have been hard to look after him with all of that going on.

Grandpa still talked frequently about leaving. At times I had the feeling that the pills we were giving him daily made him feel tired. When he felt tired, he often became desperate to "go home," which caused a vicious circle of frustration. "I'm tired. I'm going home" seemed so incongruous to us, because it meant that Grandpa would head for the door and start walking away instead of seeking rest. Now I used sterner methods of controlling him, either bolting the doors or blocking his progress so he couldn't get too far from home.

The school year ended, and Cindy began applying for part-time work wherever there was a help-wanted sign: ice cream parlors and clothing and grocery stores. Mike suggested she try the gas station where he had been working evenings. She was hired to work as a cashier in the little hut where people paid for their self-serve gasoline. She quickly learned how to make change, count her receipts, and use a measuring pole to record the amount of gas in the tanks below the ground. The gas station was close to home, so she could walk or ride her bike there and back. Like her older sisters and brothers, she would put most of the money she earned into a savings account for college. She took two weeks from her job to attend Blue Lake Fine Arts Camp in Michigan, where she lived in a communal tent and attended classes in choral singing.

Terese returned from the university, where one of her goals had been to qualify for a life-saving certificate so that when she worked as a camp counselor this summer she would be able to take her charges to the lake. She persuaded the local YMCA to sell her a short-term membership so she could continue swimming every day until June eleventh, when she would leave to go to Michigan for her second summer at the "Y" camp there.

Another goal Terese had set for herself was to go to London for the fall semester in an international student program which would enable her to study literature and drama at the University of London with a group of American students and teachers. College credit would be given from the home school. It would not advance her biology major, but it would certainly enhance her overall education. She would have a one-week break in August between her work at camp and her scheduled flight to London, with a two-week guided tour of Europe before the semester of study began. We were all very excited about Terese's adventure.

Mart was spending the summer back at the "Y" camp in northern Wisconsin, going on fishing and canoe trips with the children, teaching some classes, and doing odd jobs. Mike was busier than ever, working both at the "Y" and at the gas station for the summer, because he planned to begin a teacher-certification course at Elmhurst College in the fall. It would take two years of part-time classes to complete the program, including one semester of practice teaching. He would try to schedule his classes around his bus driving job.

Another exciting announcement came that summer: Marian and Jim were anticipating their first baby in February. It was a joyous surprise.

Milt and I celebrated our thirtieth wedding anniversary with a weekend at a chateau in Elgin, Illinois, while Marian, Pat, and baby Shawn stayed with Grandpa, with Cindy and Mike providing backup support. It was pleasant to have two whole days away by ourselves.

Grandpa's fascination with paper helped him to pass the time. We now put colorful advertising supplements from the newspaper, old catalogs, and junk mail on the table in the family room for him. These were his playthings for hours because he could no longer do more complex things.

> Meaningless papers
> in layer after layer
> carefully folded.

> Stiff fingers clutching
> or stealthily pocketing
> smeared, wrinkled treasures.

> Life's work reduced to
> a reason for being in
> fragments of junk mail.

Grandpa was sick twice during the summer, complaining of stomach pain and nausea, but each time the discomfort passed without medical assistance. I thought it was probably a gallbladder problem again, so I made sure to watch his diet more closely, especially fats and strong-flavored vegetables.

Grandpa's weakening bladder control was becoming more of a problem for me. Although he usually indicated by urgent groaning sounds when he wanted to use the bathroom, getting him there fast enough was almost impossible. I was having to change his clothing and wash it every day, sometimes more than once, besides mopping up the floor. Still, I had the idea that "diapers" were infantile, so I couldn't imagine getting them on and off Grandpa without a big fuss. Milt had no such mental block and was determined to put an end to the torment of urinary spills.

One day he came home from the drug store with a box of absorbent pads for adults. The product was both simple and effective: a large pad with button openings at the four corners, and elastic straps that buttoned on at the two sides. To my surprise, they were so easy to use that Grandpa hardly knew what was happening. While he was seated on the toilet, it was very simple to place the elastic straps, with diaper attached, around his legs, so that when he stood, pulling up the diaper was as easy as pulling up the underwear. We began using these every day, and it saved much cleanup time.

Sometimes it happened that, after Grandpa was situated in the bathroom, I would need to do something elsewhere, and the next thing I knew, he would be waddling around with his clothes around his ankles. Even worse, he sometimes pulled up his pants and fastened them, leaving underwear and diaper around his knees!

Gradually the bladder leakage became more pronounced, and we used pads with extra absorbency at night. However, Grandpa remained unpredictable. He could go as long as twelve or fourteen hours without urinating at all; or he could be in the bathroom every five minutes (or so it seemed) and have a wet pad every time.

Milt said he didn't mind changing Grandpa's wet diapers, but when he lost his bowel control, that would be the end of home care. Grandpa retained his bowel control, however, having very few accidents, even when he suffered diarrhea once or twice. We were thankful not to have this problem to deal with.

In August Milt experienced a "Rocky Mountain high" on an eight-day backpacking excursion. He and his friend Carl flew to Colorado and were joined there by a longtime camping buddy of ours, Don, who had moved to California. It seemed amazing to me that they would fly over a thousand miles to get back to the primitive life, but for Milt and his friends it was also an inward journey: a conquering of nature in order to find the inner self. Milt described sitting in camp looking out at the intense blue of a mountain lake, majestic snow-capped peaks reaching high in every direction, streams cascading down the mountainsides, and a profusion of yellow wildflowers. The quiet was profound: the stillness broken only by the trickle of water or the harsh sound of gravel underfoot. There were opportunities to be alone and to think about the meaning of life. At one point Don asked, "Why did God make all of this?"

After some thought, Milt's answer was, "So that people would turn to God to ask that very question."

My own inward journey, after Milt's return, took me back to Green Lake and the annual Christian Writers' Conference. This year there was a new poetry instructor, Lenore Coberly, a woman whose description of her work teaching creative writing to senior citizens gave me an immediate feeling of affinity. She challenged me (and the class) to make a leap through poetry from the prosaic, or commonplace, object, to where we were inside, a leap into ourselves "to find some light, some insight that we believe will burn steadily for us."

The leaps for me during that week were fantastic. I decided that, since my full-time preoccupation was with Grandpa, he would be the primary subject of my writing efforts. My first poem was "The Fire Hydrant," which expressed some of my feelings about Grandpa. A study of the Haiku form on the next day suggested "Meaningless Papers." On the third day of class, the instructor placed a number of objects on the table. We were to select one and describe it in a brief exercise. One of the objects was a short-stemmed artificial chrysanthemum made of corn husks, dyed blue, obviously very old, stuck carelessly into a hole in a dirty white shoe box. As I looked at the various objects, my eyes kept returning to that bedraggled-looking flower, and it became for me a short-stemmed red geranium picked by Grandpa and trailing petals on the floor. I knew I had the makings of a poem. That afternoon I began writing, and the words flowed through tears to the page as if memorized. I felt that the poem was good. The response of my classmates and the instructor on the next day confirmed my feeling. They suggested that I change the title (I had called it "He Brings Me Flowers") to "Alzheimer's Disease," since it was descriptive of the disease and I needed to alert the reader to that fact. (This poem appears on page 206.)

The next day's assignment led me to travel inward, not with Grandpa but with my own father. I had been devastated by his illness and death nine years before, and other attempts to write about my feelings had been futile. Now I felt a release of energy and capability within me as I strove to write a poem about him.

Again, I wrote through tears; it was a therapeutic, healing experience. This was my leap into my deepest self, in which I made a connection with my father-parent and my Father-God. For me, the writing of this poem was a significant accomplishment, and I had a moment of pride when the poem was selected as first in the contest at the end of the week.

Part of my tremendous feeling of power and success during that week was due, I believe, to the affirmation I received from my instructor and my classmates, all very competent writers. It was as if I were on a drug-induced high. Everything I wrote during that week seemed better than I had ever done before. I felt that I had been reborn as a poet, that my life would be different from that time on.

My Hand Was Small

My hand was small inside your big one.
Hopping and skipping to keep up with you,
I was impatient with your reluctance
    to supply Cheerios and Orphan Annie rings.
But you gave me books and dreams.

Then I no longer needed you.
Other hands were in mine,
    and other feet danced beside me.
Children's voices pleaded with me
    for gumballs and cowboy boots,
Yet you were always there.
I still had dreams.

I remember the call: Daddy . . . paralyzed!
Shaken, not knowing what to feel,
I wanted so much to help.
But my family, my little ones, needed me.
I served you
    by serving them.

Oh, yes, we went to visit you,
    and sat, discussing basketball.
Basketball?
Incredible, the blanket on my brain

suffocating thoughts, tears, questions
anything of import, anything of life ending,
dreams unfulfilled.

Too late, you lay, comatose.
My tears flowed freely
    at your funeral.
My brother spoke eloquently
    of your gift of love,
A gift I hadn't even noticed
    in my busy-ness, my self-absorption.

But now, confident, I soar above the din,
Reaching for heights beyond my view.
Remembering my hand in yours,
    your wisdom, fortitude,
I hear your voice within me
    comforting, challenging,
Giving me dreams.

When the conference ended and I drove home alone, I was
still in a euphoric state. I sang and talked to myself as I drove
along, and I concluded that I had enjoyed a "Rocky Mountain
high" equal to, if not surpassing, Milt's. Then I decided that, in
order to prolong his high and mine, I would throw a big surprise
birthday party for him on August twenty-eighth, which was only
two weeks away. Everyone we knew would be invited, and the
climax of the evening would be a song and dance especially for
Milt by a "Hollywood starlet"—me, in disguise.

What fun it was to actually carry out these plans in the two
weeks that followed. Milt's secretary helped with invitations, and
I contacted my sisters, neighbors, friends from church, and
friends from the school community. I hired two women I knew
from RE:AL to help in the kitchen during the party itself, planned
a simple menu, and invited people to bring a dish to share if they
wished. I also hired a group to play dance music—some young
people who played music at church and who were pleased to
entertain us for a small donation.

Milt was unaware that anything more than a small family affair
was planned for his birthday. He was incredulous when he walked

outside on the patio and saw several friends, and then more and more arriving until there were about one hundred in all. Fortunately, the weather was perfect.

My "Hollywood starlet" act made quite a hit. I wore false eyelashes and a blond wig and a sparkling outfit I had borrowed. I wrote my own song with corny rhyming verses. Cindy played guitar for me and taped me singing it—in case I had a lapse of memory in the excitement of the moment. Milt loved it.

Grandpa was oblivious to it all. My friend Jane took care of him, and he stayed inside where there was less commotion. He went to bed and slept soundly. It was a most memorable end to the summer.

My excitement over my experience at Green Lake continued. In order to find some uninterrupted time to devote to poetry, I began rising at five o'clock at least one morning every week. This gave me two extra hours in which to write, study, or just read poetry. During the day, I found other time to set about marketing the poems I had written. My instructor had suggested that I send my poems about Grandpa to the *New England Journal of Medicine*, since they had to do with Alzheimer's disease. The *Journal* sometimes published poetry, she said, and she supplied the address. I sent four poems. Within a short time, I received a letter stating that one of them, the one entitled "Alzheimer's Disease," would be included as a letter to the editor in a forthcoming issue. That was quite a thrill!

The name Alzheimer's disease, once an obscure medical term, had become a fairly common phrase in only a few years' time. My friends often remarked that it seemed that more people were "getting it" now than ever before. My own opinion, which reflected what I had read about Alzheimer's, was that the average life expectancy had risen so that there were many more older people. Moreover, as information about Alzheimer's became better known, the symptoms of Alzheimer's—failure to remember recent information, getting lost in familiar surroundings, loss of ability to work with numbers, confusion and frustration sometimes leading to extreme mood and personality changes—were more readily recognized as such. There were other diseases that resulted in similar types of dementia. However, Alzheimer's seemed now to be by far the most common of these.

The increased frequency of the diagnosis of Alzheimer's disease had led to an organized effort on the part of the families of persons afflicted with the disease to raise funds for research and to publicize the need for community support. Much had been done in the past several years. Research had revealed the content of the diseased cells and a number of possible causes for the disease. Creative efforts had been made to devise treatment methods. But much more needs to be learned before a cause is known and effective treatment can be established.

ADRDA had been working diligently on the state and national levels urging reform of government policies to address the needs of families experiencing Alzheimer's disease. Progress was sought in the areas of research, health services, training for support personnel, and tax relief.*

One evening, at a regular meeting of our ADRDA support group, the leader introduced a guest, Mr. James Vanden Bosch, a film maker who had come to ask whether any of the group members might be willing to participate in the making of a documentary film on the problems of aging. Milt asked me how I felt about it, and because of our previous good experience of sharing our story, I said I would be willing to volunteer. He gave our name and phone number to Mr. Vanden Bosch, who said he would be calling us soon.

Indeed, he did call, and we made an appointment for him to come and talk with us on a Sunday in September. He stayed for five or six hours, asking us all sorts of questions and encouraging us to share our feelings about Grandpa having Alzheimer's and about living with the day-to-day problems of dealing with Milt's dad in our family. About one week later, Jim (by now we were on a first-name basis) and his filming crew spent an evening with

*ADRDA's efforts still continue. The national *ADRDA Newsletter* (70 East Lake Street, Chicago, Illinois 60601), published quarterly, keeps members informed of the status of bills brought before the United States Congress, and regional chapter newsletters provide information on state legislation. These are valuable resources for families, enabling them to keep abreast of efforts to alleviate the special problems they face daily.

Milt, Cindy, Marian, Grandpa, and me, exploring what we were doing, why, and our feelings about it.

It was very beneficial for us to have this talk, especially for Cindy. She revealed that she had harbored a lot of resentment because of all the friction Grandpa had triggered in our family, and because of his usurping of authority over her during the first few years. The talking we did together helped me to recognize the importance of encouraging family members to express their true feelings in an open, uncritical atmosphere.

The crew returned a few days later and stayed for eight hours. While the camera rolled, Jim focused his questions on the areas we had discussed previously. He encouraged us to carry on our regular daily activities as normally as possible. He had obtained permission to photograph Grandpa and me in a grocery store we visited frequently, so we went there in the afternoon. When Cindy came home from school, she practiced her piano music. They filmed some of that—and used it as background for the intro- duction and ending of the thirty-minute film. They filmed us as we sat down to have dinner. In the evening we put Grandpa to bed (he didn't fuss that night) and then talked some more. We talked about how we felt about caring for Grandpa, how it had affected our relationships with one another and our outlook on life in general; and we described the multiple problems we had faced and were facing each day of Grandpa's interminable illness. The crew didn't leave until ten-thirty that night.

The work of completing and editing the film took months. Three other families were also studied and filmed, so that ours was only one segment of the final product. The result was an award-winning film entitled *My Mother, My Father*, that has been used by health professionals all over the country who are working with families dealing with the care of aged parents. The brochure developed to advertise the film has a picture of Grandpa on its cover.* Jim invited Milt and me and members of the other three families appearing in the documentary to attend various showings

*The same picture of Grandpa used by Terra Nova Films for the brochure from their film, *My Mother, My Father*, has been used for the jacket of this book, by permission of Terra Nova Films.

of the film and act as panel members during discussions. This, too, was a very moving experience for each of us; it convinced us even more of the powerful emotions involved in this subject, and of the need for more work and research in this area.

That fall, for an assignment in her junior English class, Cindy chose to write about Grandpa. She wrote the following story in which she describes a typical event from his point of view.

CINDY'S STORY: PRISONER OF THE MIND

"I hate you! I hate you!" I screamed at them, daring them to challenge me. Those people, they take everything I have. It's getting late and I have to be home. I go to the door, but it is locked. I can't get out. The panic rises within me as I turn to a man standing there. "I gotta go home," I tell him. He shrugs his shoulders. I try again. "It's locked. I can't get out. I have to go. It's late. I have to go home."

"I'm sorry," he says, "but you can't leave now. You can stay here. This is your home."

"Open the door!" I scream at him.

"No. I can't. You can stay here."

"I hate you!" I say again. I know he locked the door just so I couldn't get out. I can see it in his eyes. I feel my face burning with hatred, and I try the door again. It doesn't open. Maybe there's another door. I walk through the hall to look for another door. There are some papers on the table, all messed up. I have to straighten them. I put them together in neat piles. Someone comes into the room and tells me to leave his things alone. He takes the papers away from me. I try to grab them back, but I am too tired. It's late. I have to go home. I find some other papers, a spoon, and a small saucer. I will need them later. I carefully pack them up and walk to the door. I try not to let anyone see what I'm carrying. I try the door. It opens easily and I walk out. I walk to the end of the driveway and turn towards home. I have to go west. That's where my home is—west. After I have walked a short distance, there is a woman with me.

"Hello, Frank," she says.

"Go away!" I snap back. "I'm going home."

"But your home is over there." She points. I don't even bother looking. I just keep walking.

"Where are you going?" she asks.

"Home!"

"See that house over there?" she points again. I stop and look back. "The Honels live there. Is your name Honel? My name is Honel; we should stay together. Let's go this way."

She leads me back to the house, pulling my arms so that I have no choice but to go with her. I'm too tired anyway. But then I remember my wife will be waiting for me. She will get mad at me if I'm not home.

"But my wife . . ." I start to say.

"Grandpa, your wife died years ago. You live here now, with your son and his family. You stay here now."

"No," I say. My voice sounds funny, but I can't help it. My wife, dead? Years ago? "No," I say again. "She was a good woman, my wife," I tell the woman next to me. She nods her head.

"You live here now. Come on, I'll show you."

"Thank you," I say, and kiss her hand. "Thank you."

"Mom, telephone."

"Okay—you want to take Grandpa in the house?"

"Sure. Come this way, Grandpa, over here. Look! There's your room, see?"

The epilogue to Cindy's story read, "I watch as his face lights up with recognition and wonder what exactly goes on in his mind and why he thinks he must go home even though he is at home with his family. Well, at least he's not mad anymore."

It pleased me to know that Cindy was concerned enough about Grandpa to want to write about him and to try to understand why he did some of the things he did. I could see that this experience was making a deep impression on her.

During one of my early-morning writing periods, my own thoughts turned to Grandpa's habit of talking constantly: how it had revealed his feelings to us over the years, particularly now that his mind was less rational. In a study of his various moods, I wrote his words as I recalled hearing them, a kind of poetic, rhythmic flow ranging from contentment to anger and back again. As the disease progressed, this habit had become a compulsion. With each breath he would say something, usually two or three words that expressed his thoughts or feelings at that moment. If there was no particular feeling he would keep repeating "My, my." This was very annoying, but it was something we had to get used to.

Moods of Alzheimer's: Speech Patterns of a Victim

Morning

Good morning! It's nice. Very nice. I like it.
What shall I do? What shall I do? What shall I do?
Thank you. It's good. You're so good. You want to eat, too.
You take half. You have to take half! Lady, where are you?
Come here! I want to give you. Where are they? Nobody.
Nobody comes. What shall I do? I don't like it. What's this?

Oh, oohh—I feel bad. Toilet! Oh, I feel bad.
It hurts. Oohh. It hurts. Here. Something wrong.
Wait, what are you doing? What's that for?
Sit down? No, I'm afraid. Water. I don't want it.
I don't like it. I'm afraid. It's going. It's going.
It's going.

(Arranging newspapers)

What's this? My, my. My, my. My, my. My, my. My, my.
Ninety. Very nice. It'll be good. How nice. I make it.
Very nice. That's nice. For us. It be nice. Very nice . . .

Late Afternoon

Nothing. I ain't got nothing. No good. They take it.
They take everything. I'm going home. Where is it?
I don't know. I'm going. Out. I have to get out.
Let me out. God dammit. Let me out. I want out.
Bastar'! Bastar'! That's what you are. You're no good.
Let me out. I want to get out.

Evening

My, my. My, my. My, my. Come with you?
Now? Okay. My, my. My, my. My, my. My, my.
Down? Here? Lay down? Me?
My, my. My, my. My, my. My, my . . .

As each day progressed, there was a pattern of behavior that ranged from passive and contented to agitated and angry, with the agitation occurring anywhere from midafternoon through evening and sometimes into the night. At these times, nothing could satisfy Grandpa. He became so "hyper" that it was as if he were wired for electricity and the switch was on. He was on his feet constantly, moving from room to room, picking things up, tearing at them, going to the door, and going outside regardless of the weather or his state of dress; if he tried to go outside and the door wouldn't open, he would hammer on it furiously with his fist, all the while fuming and repeating "I want to go out!" and more colorful expressions.

As caretakers, each of us in the family had strong feelings of our own, running the gamut from positive to negative. Unfortunately, it was much easier to talk about the negative. It was good for us to acknowledge those feelings, yet the negatives often led to positives that we might never have experienced but for this situation.

Milt continued to take responsibility for Grandpa's calls during the night. Perhaps five or six nights out of a week, Grandpa would wake up at least once. Sometimes he went back to sleep after a trip to the bathroom, sometimes not. I found that, in spite of years of sleeping always on the alert, whether for a child's cry or Grandpa's voice, now there were many occasions when I was totally oblivious to Grandpa's calls. I had successfully unlearned the "mother instinct" response. I thanked Milt often for his help. I wanted him to know that I appreciated it.

I was still taking Grandpa with me in the car whenever I needed groceries and other supplies. One store that I visited periodically was a bulk food store. I liked to go there for special foods like granola for breakfast cereal, nuts, raisins, and other goodies to add to it, variety cheeses, bran for Grandpa's cereal, and other items. It was a small store, and there were no shopping carts; instead, we used hand baskets in which to place our purchases as we helped ourselves. At first, Grandpa held the basket for me and followed me around until I was ready to go to the cashier. This soon became tiring for him because there was nothing to lean on, so I began taking a folding chair along. I would open it up for him in an out-of-the-way place, hand him a basket to hold for me, and then go around the store to collect the items I needed, bringing each one back to him so that he would know that he was helping me. He didn't mind. It helped to pass the time. He sat there saying, "My, my."

One day when we did this, Grandpa went into one of his uncooperative moods. He didn't want to give me the basket when I was ready to leave. Realizing that I was probably going to have more problems with him, I gathered the things from the basket under his protest that I was stealing them, took them to the cashier, paid my bill, and put the bag in the car before going back for Grandpa.

As I feared, Grandpa refused to get up from the chair to come with me. I yanked him up by the arms and quickly folded the chair so he couldn't sit down again. Then I began alternately pulling and pushing him slowly down the aisle and across the middle of the store, with Grandpa becoming more and more resistant as we went along. I was trying not to draw any more attention to us than necessary, but suddenly Grandpa's knees seemed to fold slowly under him, and before I knew it he was sitting on the floor!

"My, . . . my. My, . . . my," he said, while I glared at him exasperatedly. I knew from previous experience that it was impossible for me to lift Grandpa from the floor, but now I tried, and he tried to get up, to no avail. Shoppers walked around us, looking down at him with frowns on their faces, giving me questioning glances. One woman asked if she could help.

"Thanks, but I think we'll manage," I said. I didn't know how at the moment. Other times I had summoned Milt. It wasn't that Grandpa was so terribly heavy. He probably weighed only 140 pounds. That was simply more weight than I could lift.

To his credit, Grandpa knew it was up to him. He reached

out for something to hold on to, but he was right in the middle of the aisle and couldn't reach anything. I held his hands and tugged. That didn't get him up, but it helped him scoot to where he could reach the corner of one of the cabinets that held the food bins. He reached up and was able to grasp and hold on with one hand; I lifted him from under his other arm until he could turn and get on one knee. At last he was on his feet. He shuffled willingly the rest of the way to the door and out to the car. I never took him inside that store again. Whenever I went back, either I left him in the car while I shopped, or someone stayed at home with him. I always remembered my embarrassment, and I thought everyone must recognize me and recall the strange predicament I was in that day.

There were many occasions when I needed a sitter to stay with Grandpa as fall activities enfolded. Our parish RENEW program swung into full gear with prayer meetings, planning meetings, film presentations, and potluck night planned by our committee, plus our small group meetings, all held in the evening. Besides that, as chairperson of a committee for spiritual awareness, I organized a "Day of Recollection" for the women's group. My friend Ann stayed with Grandpa on that day, and when I returned I saw the two of them down at the end of the block. With them was our wheelchair—the one we had bought second-hand in case we'd need it for Grandpa. We had never used it, but kept it handy simply because there was no place to store it. Ann was trying to convince Grandpa to sit down in the chair so that she could get him back home. I commended her for her creative problem solving. It worked—finally.

A friend from RE:AL called one day and invited me to join a writers' group that met monthly in the homes of members. Two of the members were people I knew from RE:AL, and all had published writings of some kind. I was honored to be included in the group. They called themselves the "Scribblers."

Milt was involved not only in the RENEW activities with me but also in his many school-affiliated activities. One of these necessitated his presence at the school each Saturday morning from September through April as part of a "French Back-to-Back" program. A group of fifth-graders from our school district was being prepared for a two-week trip to France which would take place in May. Similarly, a group of French children would visit our schools in March. This program was strictly voluntary, and all expenses were paid by the parents of the children involved. However, an administrator had to be in charge each year, and now it was Milt's turn. Because the administrator had to donate much of his time, the school district offered him the chance to go to France for one week while the children were there. Milt was definitely planning to go. He insisted that I go with him (at our expense, of course). This was such an unusual opportunity that I hoped to find some way to arrange it.

Milt was also excited about the new availability of computers. He was taking an evening course in computer basics and struggled with learning the new "language." He shared his enthusiasm with the other school administrators and with his teachers. When the district purchased computers for the use of the elementary-school children, Milt's school was the first in the district to set up a class schedule so that all the teachers and students could become familiar with the new technological marvel. He held what he called a "Traveling Road Show," in which ten available computers were brought to his school for one week so that ten children could have hands-on experience at the same time. In the evening, parents were invited to do the same.

Meanwhile, our letters from Terese were filled with her enthusiasm for the great treasures of Europe. She traveled briefly to France, Belgium, and Holland and then settled in England, where she studied literature, drama, and culture, attending many plays and venturing around London by way of the "tube," as well as making some excursions into the countryside. During the midterm break she traveled alone to Ireland, where she met and stayed with some of my mother's cousins, experiencing her "roots," for five wonderful days.

I realized how far away Terese was when my letters didn't reach her for six days, and it took more than two weeks to receive an answer to a question. We missed her particularly on Thanksgiving Day, when all the rest of the family shared our turkey dinner. Little Shawn, now seven months old, sat in the old high chair that all six of our children had used, munching rolls and crackers. We turned on the tape recorder after dinner to make a recording for Terese. Nobody could think of anything to say, so there was a hodge-podge of sound: Shawn's gurgling and giggles, several conversations going on at once, and Grandpa's monologue in the background. I decided to focus on one subject, and all I could think of was something that had been preying on my mind. So I said, "Your dad and I have talked about what we will do when Grandpa dies, as far as what kind of funeral he should have, and I was wondering what all of you think about this."

Pat: Grandpa should have just a regular funeral like everybody else, shouldn't he?

Marian: Certainly. Whatever's customary.

Milt: Can any of you remember Babi's funeral?

Marian: I do, sort of. There was this weird guy who talked in Bohemian.

Milt: That's right. There was no church service, just a short talk in Bohemian and then in English by someone hired by the funeral home. That was the way Grandpa wanted it.

Pat: Yeah, and we never went to the cemetery!

Rosalie: Well, we went first to the funeral home and then to a sort of chapel at the cemetery. I remember they asked us ahead of time whether we wanted to go to the grave site or not, and I think we just decided not to. Then afterward we had a hard time locating the grave when we went back to see it and to arrange for the stone.

Pat: I don't like that at all. I think we should go to the cemetery, and I think there should be a Mass, too.

Cindy: Yeah, I think so, too.

Marian: You know I'm not great on going to church, but if church is important at all, it should be when someone dies.

Milt: I disagree. I don't think we should have a Mass for Dad because he never believed in church. He used to ridicule me when I went as a kid.

Marian: Oh, oh, I detect some buried hostility here, huh, Dad?

Milt: You're right. We used to argue about religion all the time, and he embarrassed me in front of my friends. He never went to church, and my mother only went on Christmas and Easter. But she encouraged me to go.

Mart: Don't you think it would be okay for Grandpa now? I mean that was a long time ago.

Mike: Wait a minute. Who's the Mass for—the person that died or the people who go to it?

Rosalie: Both, really.

Mike: Then Grandpa should have a Mass and everything, just like if one of us died.

Pat: Yeah, I think so, too. After all, he's our grandfather, and our friends and relatives will probably be there.

Marian: Yes, the wake and the funeral service and all that are for the family. It's very important to do that together.

Mike: Grandpa is more Christian than a lot of people I know. He was always good to us. I feel that Grandpa has learned things since he has been with us. I didn't believe he had Alzheimer's disease, but now I guess he does have it, and maybe for him it was a good thing that he got it. I mean, it made him see that sometimes a person has to give up and let go. I've learned a lot from him. I know he wants things his way pretty much; that's why he always wants to go home. He never wanted to come here. Why should he? At home he could be alone with his flowers, eat whatever he wanted, do whatever he wanted. He comes here and we're always telling him what he can't do, what he can't eat, and where he can't go—or else we ignore him completely, like right now.

Grandpa's voice could be heard from the family room, where he sat fiddling with his papers, saying, "My, my. My, my. . . . I can't. I can't make it. My, my. I want to go someplace. I don't feel so good. Oh . . . ohhh . . ."

Milt: I'll take him to the bathroom.

Rosalie: Okay. I agree, Mike. I think a Catholic funeral would be appropriate for Grandpa when he dies.

Everyone was silent for a while.

Milt returned to the living room after a few minutes. "You know, you're right. You've all helped me to see that what happened in the past has nothing to do with it. Dad is part of my family now, and church is very much a part of our lives, so Grandpa should have a church service and a Catholic burial."

Rosalie: Good! I'm glad that's settled, even though it probably won't happen for a long time.

Cindy: Hey, the tape recorder is still on. Is this for Terese, too?

Rosalie: Sure, why not? Let's all sing a song for Terese. What song can we sing?

Cindy: How about 'Happy Thanksgiving to You,' to the tune of 'Happy Birthday'?

Milt: [beginning to sing] Hap-py Thanks-giv-ing to you, . . ."

Everyone joined in, while Mart picked up Shawn and set him on the piano bench. He added his pounding on the keys to finish the song with a flourish. Everybody had a good laugh.

Terese returned from London in Mid-December. Milt, Cindy, and I picked her up at the airport, and Marian came over after work that evening. The five of us sat around the kitchen table asking questions and attempting to fill in the gaps caused by Terese's absence. Grandpa also sat at the table with us, a loud presence demanding attention, causing lapses in the conversation as phrases were drowned out, repeated, and drowned out again. Cindy fetched Grandpa's doll. It was a little, plastic, red-haired doll that had been put away in her closet years ago. Marian had ferreted it out for Grandpa when she had stayed here with him recently.

"What a good idea! I would never have thought of that," said Terese, as Grandpa looked intently at the doll and touched its face with his finger. He was silent for a while, as the conversation resumed. Then his voice boomed again:

"My, my. I got this to do. . . . I can't get it out. . . . I'm, put this in here . . . Over here!" He indicated he wanted Cindy to do something with the doll, but she didn't understand what he wanted her to do. "What you got . . . here . . . already . . . this one . . . My, my. Here . . . I try . . . I like to make that . . . I gotta make it like . . . You don't care. . . . I wish I would have it. . . . Look at that. . . . I'm trying . . . all this. . . ."

While he was talking, the rest of us were all trying to talk and listen at the same time, rather unsuccessfully. Grandpa was poking the doll and pulling its arm. Milt said, "Ouch!" Everybody laughed.

"Somebody gotta do it," Grandpa continued, now pulling the doll's hair. "All right, go ahead . . . you like something, go ahead. I got no time. I got work here to do. You hear me?" He stood up and shuffled into the family room.

Did he think we were laughing at him? I wondered what it was like to be unable to understand what was being said, to have thoughts and be unable to communicate them clearly, to hear laughter and wonder: What was the joke I missed? Are they laughing at me?

Terese quizzed her sister Marian, now in her seventh month of pregnancy. "Is the baby kicking? Can I feel it? Do you think it's a girl or a boy? What names have you picked?"

She shared some of her observations about the British people: "I never saw an overweight person the whole time!" "They take their dogs everywhere. Even on the trains. They never bark or anything. I couldn't believe it! We rode the 'tube' everywhere. You didn't need a car at all. It was great, even late at night, and we were never afraid of getting mugged. It was perfectly safe!" She expressed the embarrassment she had felt when London headlines mocked the American furor over Cabbage Patch dolls. She had made new friends. She had enjoyed an exciting time abroad. Soon she would return to the ordinary life of a student at Western Illinois University.

Also in mid-December, I found a new source of excitement in the publication of my poem "Alzheimer's Disease" in the *New England Journal of Medicine*. I hadn't heard anything more about it until the telephone rang one afternoon. It was a call from a woman in Ohio who had just read my poem in her husband's magazine and liked it so much that she phoned to tell me. I was completely overwhelmed! It was a beautiful feeling to hear this person I had never met describe the emotion she felt as she read about my experience and related it to her own, which was working with geriatric patients in horticulture therapy (something I had never even heard of). I was thrilled to think that what I had shared had made a difference to her.

Alzheimer's Disease*

On summer days
He walks or sits outside to pass the hours
    empty, monotonous hours—
    weeks and months of present moments,
    hollow moments.
His eye may catch upon a misplaced garden tool
    perhaps an empty flower pot, discarded,
    or a branch blown by a recent storm.
Carefully he places them just so,
    or brings them in,
    to guard them from the grasp of thieves.
He may walk around the fenced-in garden,
    becoming caught in chicken-wire and compost,
    green tomatoes tempting,
And red geraniums.
The brilliant flower clusters call
    some earlier day perhaps
    when, time-laden,
    he sprouted them and nurtured them through winter
    in rusted tin-can pots.
Geraniums, so radiant of hue,
    he bends arthritic hips and knees,
    defying loss of balance,
    drawn by hypnotic color
    selecting, choosing
    this one.
To the door he shuffles
    opening carefully, slowly,
    grasping frame with one hand,
    flower in the other,
    studying through blurred vision as he
    steps, up, over
    into the house.

*First published in the *New England Journal of Medicine*, 309 (15 December 1983): p. 1524. Permission granted to reprint.

Traumatic for geranium petals
  they float gently down,
  under his feet, leaving
  walked-on stains of red
  here and there.
    Here's something
    something good.
    You take it.
His demand sets me on edge;
  seeing red marks on the floor
  I want to say, "Don't pick the geraniums,"
  and then I know,
He's just a two-year-old,
  bringing me flowers.

After that, I began getting letters in response to the poem from people all over the United States and Canada and even from Europe. Some were forms requesting copies for reference. Some contained personal stories of Alzheimer's patients who were either spouses or parents of the letter-writers (many of whom were doctors). Invariably they thanked me for sharing my experience.

I especially enjoyed a telephone call from a doctor in Kentucky. He said that he really liked my poem and that it brought back memories of time spent working in a Veterans Administration hospital years ago. He said I seemed to have a great knowledge about Alzheimer's (!), so I told him that I had received one curt response from a doctor who said that what I had described was not Alzheimer's at all. He laughed and said that he had thought I might be a neurologist! That was amusing to me, but apparently the majority of people who publish in and read the *Journal* are in the medical profession. Anyway, we had a nice chat. What a thrill it was to be able to touch people so remote from me!

The Midwest suffered a deep freeze at Christmas that year, causing many cars to be temporarily inoperative. Marian phoned on the afternoon of the holiday to say that both her car and Jim's were frozen, and they couldn't join us for dinner unless someone would pick them up.

Mart volunteered. He had just returned from a church service at the United Pentecostal Church. (He was a recent convert to the denomination in Green Bay and had located a similar church in a nearby suburb through scanning the Yellow Pages.)

No one mentioned going to the nursing home to sing carols. Our disrupted experience of last year had diminished our enthusiasm for the project—or maybe it had somehow served its purpose for us. This was Shawn's first Christmas, and that was quite enough excitement added to the gift exchange. His little face shone with curiosity at the sparkling lights and ornaments on the tree and all the brightly wrapped packages, many of them for him to tear open.

The cold weather continued, but Milt and Mike packed their woolens, boots, and skis and headed for Wisconsin on the day after Christmas, providing Mart with a ride back to Green Bay and his job as a janitor's helper at the YMCA. The two of them visited the family Mart was rooming with, stayed overnight, and drove further north the next day. They put up their tent in a campground and cooked a quick dinner after dark, with the temperature at three degrees. Once in their tent and arctic sleeping bags, they were able to sleep comfortably. Skiing was good in the midday sunshine, but the next night the temperature dropped to the minus twenties. Fortunately they had contacted my elderly aunt who lived in the area. She insisted they camp in her living room that night, which they did. The next day it was too cold to ski, so after a hearty lunch they packed up and drove for some seven hours to get home.

As New Year's Day came around, I made a resolution to try a new approach to Grandpa's care. Four years ago, I had taken Grandpa to a day care center in Elmhurst, just briefly, to see how it might compare with the one in Cicero. I found that it had even less staff, and I could see that there was no way for Grandpa to fit into their program. But he had changed quite a bit since that time. The topic of day care was a popular one at our ADRDA support group meetings. It had worked out beautifully for several members of the group. Even though my previous experiences— both in Cicero and in Elmhurst—had indicated that Grandpa was too hard to manage, I began thinking about it again. He was considerably more passive and quiet than he had ever been. He could sit and do nothing for a couple of hours at a time. Maybe it was time to give day care another try. I telephoned the place in Elmhurst and made arrangements to take Grandpa there on Thursday after the New Year's holiday. I explained to the director that he had Alzheimer's disease, and she told me that they had several other clients with the disease. She suggested that I bring Frank at eleven o'clock so he could stay for lunch. I hoped that Grandpa would just sit quietly there, as he did much of the time at home now, and watch whatever was going on. I thought it would be good for him to be with people.

The morning was cold, crisp, and bright. Grandpa had his breakfast and sat quietly, arranging his papers. At ten-thirty, I took him to the bathroom. Then:

"Grandpa, I have to go someplace, and I want you to come with me."

"Me? Go with you? Okay."

He was in a calm, acquiescent mood. I helped him with his scarf and coat, buttoned his coat, and put a stocking cap on his head. The car was just outside the door.

"Oh! Cold!" he said.

"Yes," I said, nodding in agreement.

He followed me gingerly around to the open car door and stepped inside, left foot first, holding on to the seat with one hand and the door with the other, falling heavily once he knew the seat was under him. Then he drew his right foot stiffly inside and I closed the door.

He sat silently as we drove along.

"Grandpa, sing." I said, adding, in Bohemian, "Spee-vay." He didn't respond. I sang a few bars of "Jingle Bells" very slowly to start him out. He joined in, but soon lapsed into silence again.

We arrived at the church where the day care program was held, and went inside. The director greeted us and showed me where to put Grandpa's things. I helped him take off his coat and cap.

The director spoke to him. "Frank, you can come with me. I'd like to show you what we do here." She took his hand and he followed her, while I explained that I would return in about an hour to see how he was doing. Then, if he was okay, he could stay longer.

What a dreamer I am!

When I returned, the director expressed her relief at seeing me. She had Grandpa sitting in an armchair in the lounge, alone. The other clients were all in the dining room. Frank had been very uncooperative and disruptive, she said, and had begun taking the tableware from the table. "I'm afraid I'll have to ask you to take Frank home," she said. "He is just too difficult to handle. We don't have anyone who could stay with him, one on one. I'm sorry."

Meanwhile, Grandpa was oblivious to all that she was saying. He was playing with the remaining food on his plate. I got his coat, and the director took his food tray. He wouldn't give her his spoon.

He refused to get up. Finally I persuaded him, but he was reluctant to let me put his coat on him, or to let me button it. I got the spoon away from him, the coat on, and beckoned him to follow me. He refused. There was a long hall leading to the exit, and he would not walk. I had to resort to standing behind him, grasping his two upper arms firmly, and shoving him forward with one knee, so that he had no choice but to keep moving. No one offered to help me with him. Somehow I got the door open and pushed him through it. We still had some distance to go to the car. Since he refused to move, he had to be pushed all the way to the curb. Then he had sense enough to seek safety and held onto the car to step down. He got into the car willingly.

After we got home, I found another spoon in his pocket.

This experience was very traumatic for Grandpa. He was visibly agitated for two or three hours afterward and then became depressed.

I realized that I should not have left him alone in a strange place. Like a two-year-old left abruptly in a room full of people, he was totally confused and frustrated. Reverting to his survivor instinct, he tried to gather his "possessions" and withdraw to the security within himself.

Grandpa and I had both flunked "Day Care 101." For me, the way to share the burden of Grandpa's care was to continue to have others come to our home. There, at least, he felt secure among familiar surroundings.

Responses to my poem kept coming every few days, encouraging me to persevere with my writing. I began to think that perhaps a book format would be possible, so I decided to record as much as I could about our family's experiences. In order to do that, I would have to devote more of my time to writing. Since the day care center hadn't worked out, I asked Jane to come one afternoon each week while I went to the library to write. I found that the time spent there in the quiet room, away from the phone and other distractions of home, was most productive. Jane's manner with Grandpa was very sweet. Sometimes she hovered over him more than he liked, but they were quite used to one another. I knew that when Jane was there, I could walk away and, no matter what happened, she could handle it. What a great feeling that was!

One day I asked Jane if she would be willing to take the job of staying with Grandpa for the week in May when Milt and I wanted to go to France. We would need twenty-four-hour care. Mike was too busy with his college classes and part-time job. He simply couldn't do it, and I didn't ask him.

Jane replied that she wouldn't do the job alone, but perhaps a friend would do it with her—one in the daytime, one at night. This sounded like a good arrangement to me. She asked her friend about it, and soon we set a date to meet together and talk further.

Jane and her friend Annette stopped by on a Sunday afternoon so that Annette could meet Grandpa and our family and decide whether she would accept the job. She would. We discussed salary and agreed without difficulty on a fair amount. I could hardly believe our good fortune!

In the weeks that followed, Annette came to stay with Grandpa a number of times so that they could become better accustomed to one another. She worked as a registered nurse during the day but lived alone and supplemented her income by taking occasional jobs of this type. I was thankful to have found her. As we cared for Grandpa, it seemed that at each step of the way there was a continual process of doors closing and opening: difficulties, opportunities, obstacles, solutions. Some people might see this as coincidence. My faith told me that my family and I were receiving grace to do the job we had to do. We kept an open attitude, constantly receptive to new ideas, optimistic about finding solutions to our problems, and supportive of one another. Somehow we found everything we needed.

Although things did work out well for us, we never knew when, in a moment of frustration, Milt or I would lose our temper. Mealtime was as likely a time as any. . . .

One day Grandpa had snacked quite a bit while I was cooking dinner (he had been restless and "going home," so I had supplied him with food to distract him). Naturally, when the family assembled for the meal, he was not very hungry. He finished his soup, however, and I gave him a plate of food. He reached for a knife or fork from Milt's place, and Milt instinctively pounced on it to prevent his getting it.

Grandpa talked loudly as he toyed with his food. "My, my. My, my." We tried to carry on a normal conversation, breaking off periodically during his loud phrases, then resuming. This had become routine with the four of us at home now.

Grandpa finished half the food on his plate and began spooning the rest into his soup bowl. Then he picked up the soup bowl and dumped the food back onto the plate. Milt and I were aware of what he was doing, but, being used to it, we let him "play."

Perhaps Grandpa was feeling bored and ignored. At any rate, he got up to leave. He placed the empty soup bowl on his plate next to the food and picked up the two dishes with one hand. As he turned to move away from the table, taking the dishes with him, the plate was at an angle pointing toward the floor.

Milt tried to grab the plate. Grandpa resisted. A momentary struggle ensued, and the food ended up on the chair and on the floor.

Suddenly infuriated, Milt gave Grandpa a whack on the bottom of his pants as if he were a small child, and shoved him down on another chair. A sudden hush followed.

I handed Milt some paper towels, and he wiped up the mess, while Grandpa sat, sulking.

By this time we were finished eating anyway, so I busied myself at the sink, and Milt and Cindy loaded the dishwasher. Mike went upstairs to his room. Grandpa continued to sulk. Later

I noticed Cindy standing next to Grandpa, rubbing his back and wordlessly giving him comfort.

That evening I asked Cindy about how she felt when she did that. She replied that she had felt sorry because Grandpa didn't mean to do anything bad and he was being punished. She said that she used to like to kneel by Grandpa, lean her head against him, and pat him, but "he doesn't want me to do that anymore, so I just ignore him." This time he seemed to appreciate her loving concern.

Later that evening I had to go to a meeting. Milt stayed with Grandpa, having a chance to counter his earlier impatience and to minister to him in a loving way. After having lived with Grandpa all this time, Milt had come to see the wisdom of gentler handling, while Mike sometimes had to admit that a strong tactic like bolting the doors was the only effective one.

Our activities with the RENEW program at church were on-going and highly satisfying. People were becoming more comfortable with discussing their beliefs and with praying spontaneously, things the average Catholic had not been accustomed to doing. Those of us involved in the leadership of the program were inspired to continue planning and providing new opportunities for a deepening of faith experience for our fellow parishioners.

It would have been impossible for me to participate in these plans without the help of Jane and Ann and now Annette, who were my dependable sitters. Without their cheerful willingness to spend several hours at a time giving us respite, caring for Grandpa would have been a most confining task indeed.

On the twenty-ninth day of February, leap year day, our daughter, Marian, gave birth to our second grandson, Eric. Milt and I were privileged to visit them at the hospital that same evening in the birthing room, a room like a large bedroom where Jim had stayed with Marian throughout her labor and delivery. New life is such a miracle! We were filled with gratitude that a healthy baby had come into the world.

During the second week of March, according to schedule, twenty-five French children, part of the "French Back-to-Back" program, arrived in Elmhurst, starting a steady round of day and evening activities at school. There were three adults traveling with the children: one counselor, a woman fluent in both English and French; a French classroom teacher; and his wife. All these people were welcomed into homes in the Elmhurst school community. In order to enhance the group's visit to America, many group activities were planned either by a parent committee or by the host families. Milt, as principal of the host school, was actively involved in many of the functions, and he urged me to line up evening sitters for Grandpa so that I, too, could get to know the team—the adults, both French and American, who were involved in the program. There was a welcoming potluck at the school, organized by the parents of the American children. There were private dinner parties given by some of the host families, to which Milt and I, as well as the team, were invited. Milt asked if we could host the team for dinner at our home one evening, and we did so. There was an open house at the home of the American teacher who would be going to France with our children in May, and a team "Night on the Town" in Chicago—all of which we attended during the two-week period. The closing activity was a musical program presented by the two groups of children for the entire host school and that evening for parents, friends, and all who wanted to attend. I had been hesitant to do all this at the start, but by the time it was over I could see the wisdom of making the effort, as American citizens, to help entertain these visitors to our country—to extend our friendship to them. Naturally the subject of Alzheimer's disease came up, and it was obvious that the people in France are as concerned about the problem of Alzheimer's disease care as we are in the United States.

Terese came home for a spring break from Western Illinois University while some of the "French Back-to-Back" activities were going on, and she noticed that I was hiring sitters to watch Grandpa. "How come you don't ask Cindy and Mike to watch Grandpa anymore?" she wanted to know.

I explained that I had a different attitude about it now; that Cindy and Mike were helpful in many ways, but that I found it best to hire sitters whenever I could, to minimize depending on family too much.

"Well, you can ask me to do it while I'm here," she said. "It's hard for me to take care of Grandpa now because he can't have fun anymore. So I need to be asked. I need extra motivation to pay attention to him now." She found that he had changed profoundly while she was away. It occurred to me that Milt and I were in a similar situation. If we had not been forced to take care of Grandpa, we would have been unaware of his needs, unaware of the plight of the aged to a great extent, unaware of Alzheimer's disease and the difficulties of families caring for its victims. It is only through this difficult trial that our eyes and hearts have been opened.

Grandpa had entered another new phase. Now he seemed to need more sleep. He would wake up at eight o'clock—or else he'd still be asleep at nine in the morning, and I'd wake him. Then, instead of being alert, he would sit and drowse in his chair, uninterested in food, the balloon game, or anything else. I would try taking him for a short walk; he would be too tired. When I put him on the toilet he would fall asleep there, too.

Suddenly, in the afternoon, he would change and become restless, hungry, and hyper. He'd eat everything I brought him and want more, until finally he couldn't eat any more and started playing with the food. Then he would be on his feet, declaring he was leaving, going to the door, back to the kitchen, back to the door again, in and out of the bathroom countless times in a maze of nonstop motion.

Meanwhile, I would be trying to prepare dinner with all of this going on. Then the rest of the family would return home, and we would assemble at the table. Grandpa would talk in his loud, rhythmic fashion "My, my. What's that? . . . I do it. . . . Look here. . . . I like it. . . ." on and on while he toyed with his food, the rest of us vainly trying to carry on a conversation.

After a while Grandpa would announce again that he was "going home . . . Goodbye," and everyone would want to applaud! When he actually went outside, no one would make a move to stop him.

A minute or so later, Milt would go after him and either help him back inside or leave him out there, looking at something or walking slowly to the other entrance. In and out again he'd go, regardless of cold spring winds.

After perhaps an hour or more, he would be calm, worn out, sitting with eyes drooping again. He'd eat his supper, but when it was time to go to bed, he would refuse. "You go!" he'd say angrily to me. He would make excuses not to lie down: "My shoes are dirty." He wouldn't take them off or let me do it. "I might fall asleep." (He didn't want to sleep—who knows why!)

I would give him his pill in a bite of banana and lift his legs so he would lie down. Then I would hold his hands to comfort him a while, with the light off. At first he would breathe audibly, quickly, and I could tell he was still hyper. Gradually his breathing would become quieter, and I would tell him, "Goodnight. I'll see you in the morning," and leave the room. Usually he remained in bed. Not always.

We noticed a change in his bladder control also. We now had to change his pads three or four times a day and bought heavier ones for night use.

Also in March, one of our regular ADRDA support group meetings became rather special. It happened that the mother of one of our members had died after having suffered from Alzheimer's disease for many years. Our group leader invited other members whose loved ones had died, who no longer ordinarily attended the group meetings, to talk about their experiences with the rest of the group. It was a very moving exchange for me, and I recorded from memory some of the thoughts that were shared that night. (Names are fictitious.)

Beth, a young single woman, spoke of her father's death: "I'm glad, you know, that he's gone. I'm glad to come in from work and not see him, the way he was. But it's hard, too, because I hardly have any friends left. And now I've no excuse to stay home on a Friday night. People don't understand," she continued. "They think they do, but right away they start telling you how they felt and what happened to them. They don't want to listen to me, how I feel."

Geri spoke of her mother. "I'm not sorry; I'm relieved. At

least, now she has peace. I don't want people to tell me they're sorry. But there is a loss."

Jeanette added, "After they're gone, you remember all the good things about them. You forget the bad things, how hard it was. But you have all this time, and you don't know what to do with it. Time to think . . ."

Geri said, "It's something I wished for every day. Now I'm just glad it's over. But I keep remembering. . . ."

Jim, Geri's husband, said, "We had everything in locked drawers and cupboards. Now I know the paper towels are back on the rack where they belong, but every time I want one I reach for the drawer where we used to keep them."

Mary commented, "They're so dependent on you, and every moment of the day you're thinking about them, and then all of a sudden they're not there anymore, and you have nothing to do."

Finally Beth said, "It's good to be able to come here and know that people do understand. I feel that I can express myself without fear that I'll be taken the wrong way. The others in my family— most of them I can't even talk to yet. They're struggling with their guilt. Or jealousy. I was here. I lived with it. They didn't. I saw what needed to be done."

In April, our family happenings were Shawn's first birthday party and Eric's christening. Grandpa stayed at home with Jane or Annette. I began to wonder what I had ever done without them. I had been following Milt's suggestion and paying them by check so that I would have a record of the amount at the end of the year. He thought he might be able to include this cost on our income tax return.

Paying for this custodial care was not nearly as difficult for us as finding people to do it had been. Grandpa's social security check and pension were ample to cover all of our expenses in taking care of him at home. I paid slightly more than minimum wage to the sitters. For a few hours at a time it was reasonable, and for me it was well worth the expenditure.

Early in May, a group of twenty-two Elmhurst children departed for France with a teacher, Caroline (who was from Milt's school), and a counselor, Mike, a young man who had learned French while on a year's trip abroad. He was looking forward to a free trip to France and a chance to visit friends there, in return for his services as translator and counselor to the children in case of loneliness or other problems. Milt wished them "bon voyage" as they left with identically marked luggage and great excitement at seeing their new French friends again and flying "alone" for the first time. One week later, it was our turn to leave for France. I had written pages of directions for Jane and Annette, telling them where to find things and describing procedures. I was confident that Grandpa would get along just fine with them.

Milt and I had a comfortable flight and were met at the French airport by our friends Caroline and Mike and by Madame Claudette (a fictitious name), principal of the host school in France. She and Milt had corresponded, with the help of translators, and she had graciously provided her apartment in the city of Saint-Germain-en-Laye, a suburb about thirty kilometers (or approximately nineteen miles) from Paris, for our use during our week in France. The French government customarily provides lodging close to the schools for the teachers and principals, but Madame had a home within commuting distance of her school and used the apartment only on occasions when she had to be at school late in the evening. Therefore she made it available to us, free of charge.

We had a wonderful week. The French people demonstrated their generous hospitality, warmth, and graciousness. We were invited out to dinner twice, to lunch five times—three of those lunches were really multi-course dinners—and once to tea. We tasted all sorts of wine, often a different one with each course; numerous varieties of cheese; and delicious hard-crust bread.

Madame Claudette, with her daughter and son-in-law, took us to see the sights of Paris—the Eiffel Tower, the Versailles palace, the Cathedral of Notre Dame—and to Giverny, the city where the artist Monet's home and gardens have been restored to their original beauty. On another day we had a chance to travel to Paris by ourselves, using the *metro*, or suburban train system, and to try to shop knowing neither the language nor the money system. People were very patient and helpful. One day we traveled with both the French and American groups of children via super-fast train to the ancient city of Lyon for a guided tour of the restored historical buildings dating back to the Middle Ages. We attended the closing program presented by the American and French children for a large number of French parents, families, and friends. We were very proud of the fine representation of American culture that was given by our children. Finally, we were bused along with them to the airport for the eight-and-one-half-hour flight back to Chicago, exhausted but exhilarated by our experience.

Mike, Cindy, Jane, and Annette welcomed us back enthusiastically. Everything had gone well, and Grandpa was just the same. The two women had taken care of all the little crises that had arisen. Mike and Cindy had managed to follow a normal routine. Terese had returned from college in a frenzy of unpacking, sorting, and repacking and had left the next day for her summer-camp counseling job, two days before we got back. On Memorial Day weekend I made a "French feast" for the family, an attempt to emulate the multi-course, extravagant cuisine with which we had been feted while in France. Our sixth year of caring for Grandpa proved that we could do our best for him and at the same time pursue a fairly normal life for ourselves—with all its peaks and valleys, its stumbling and falling, its getting up and continuing the climb.

10 · The Seventh Year: Journey's End

It's a quarter past ten on a warm spring morning, and Grandpa and I are in the car on the way to his regular appointment with his urologist, Dr. Novak. These appointments come every three to four months. Grandpa is quiet as we drive, though occasionally he comments: "You are good. You know how to do it. You know everything."

We arrive at the medical building, and I park in front, using the flashing emergency signal while I get him out of the car and into the building where there is a bench to sit on. He sits down, and I caution him to stay there until I come back.

There is no designated parking for this building. I have to park along the street, one block away. When I return, he is still seated on the bench, but he is scowling.

"Thank you for waiting, Grandpa; come with me now."

"Do it yourself. I'll stay here," he answers, with a sweeping gesture of his arm.

"We can go now, Grandpa, come on. Up!"

Reluctantly, with a scornful look, he allows me to help him to his feet. Holding both his hands, I walk backwards to the elevator, where a man holds the elevator doors open for us. Grandpa shuffles inside and grasps the hand bar.

We arrive at the third floor and move slowly toward the doctor's office, passing a drinking fountain where I stop to have a drink. "Would you like a drink of water?"

He doesn't even answer. He is still scowling.

We enter the waiting room, and the receptionist tells me to take Grandpa inside. He sees the chairs and begins to sit down.

"No, Grandpa, this way." I take both hands firmly and tug, getting the message through to him. I am grateful that we do not have to wait.

The receptionist offers me a cup to take Grandpa's urine sample, but I say, "I think he's too agitated for that today."

"That's okay," she says. We proceed slowly through the short hallway to the examining room as Dr. Novak enters.

"Sit down here, Grandpa," I say, indicating the examining table. I steer him to it while unbuttoning and unzipping his pants at the same time, so that it's done by the time he is ready to sit.

The doctor speaks in a friendly manner to him in Bohemian. They used to joke back and forth with one another years ago. Now Grandpa answers gruffly, in English, "I don't want it." He repeats this several times, while the doctor and I try to coax him to lie down, to no avail.

Dr. Novak brings some lollipops, unwraps one, and sticks it in Grandpa's mouth. Then he raises the leg-rest, forcing Grandpa to lean back. I support him as he goes down, placing the waiting pillow under shoulders and head.

I hold his hands and lean over to reassure him, as Dr. Novak injects an anesthetic into his penis. Grandpa winces and flails out with his arms, but I hold them down firmly, speaking to him gently. "It's okay, Grandpa, hang on, the doctor is going to check you over. You'll be all right."

The doctor waits to be sure the anesthetic has taken effect. Then he proceeds to force tubes of successively larger diameter through the penis opening, dilating the opening and loosening the stricture. Grandpa's eyes are closed, his lips firmly sealed around the lollipop. In spite of the anesthetic, he indicates his discomfort and struggles to get free.

Finally, the procedure is finished, the spilled urine is wiped away, and Grandpa is helped to a sitting position. He is silent, the sucker still clamped tightly between his lips.

After I pull up his clothing, the doctor gives me a prescription to prevent infection. I take Grandpa to a chair in the waiting room while I write a check and make a new appointment. He is still looking sullen, angry.

"We can go home now, Grandpa."

"Never mind. I'll stay here."

"No, you can get up now. Up!" Again, I tug at his hands, and after a few more refusals he allows himself to be helped up. Slowly we work our way to the door. I am conscious of stares from others in the room.

"Go on, I'll go myself. Go on!" he says, angrily.

He follows me to the elevator and into the vestibule. Again, I must ask him to wait while I get the car. There is no one else around. He sits down.

"I'll be right back, Grandpa; you wait." He waves me away with a scornful gesture.

I hurry to the car, drive back, and park in front with the emergency signal. Again, Grandpa is reluctant to get up, but eventually he comes along with me.

Once in the car, he flings the sucker onto the dashboard in disgust. All the way home he sits, sullen; eyes narrow slits, toothless mouth shut tight.

As I drive, I am thinking about what has just happened, pleased that it went well, relieved that I don't have to worry about this for another three months, feeling competent.

I glance sideways at him, seeing him jostled by the bumps in the road, still wearing his hostile expression.

"I don't blame you for feeling bad, Grandpa. Sometimes we have to take it. The doctor helps you to stay well. But it's no fun!"

He makes no response, so I don't know whether he understands. Suddenly I see through his eyes this small incident, one among many that occur regularly in his confused, dependent, vulnerable existence. It is as if Grandpa has just been raped.

We arrive back home and return to our routine. I take Grandpa to the bathroom, seat him, and remove the gauze bandage held loosely to his penis with a rubber band. He urinates. "It hurts," he tells me.

"I know, Grandpa. I'm sorry. It'll get better."

He forgets about it quickly as he enjoys some bread and jelly soaked in milk while I prepare his lunch.

The changes in Grandpa over the six-year period of his stay with us had been so gradual as to be almost imperceptible. Looking back, however, it was easy to mark the deterioration that had taken place, both mental and physical. When Milt and I returned from France after being away for nine days, Grandpa gave no sign of recognition; he knew us no more and no less. There was a slight deterioration in his bladder control. Jane and Annette reported that he had wet the bed and his clothing several nights, in spite of the diaper pad. He was quite sedentary during the day, sometimes wetting through his pad and his clothes. Now I would have to remember to take him to the washroom more often, not waiting for him to indicate his discomfort.

Grandpa seemed to walk more slowly, too, with greater effort and fear of falling. When I wanted him to hurry (an impossibility) I would take hold of each hand and tug, his solid hulk inching forward as if he weighed a ton. I thought I might have to stop taking him to the grocery store with me. Twice he dragged his feet and was uncooperative.

It was eight o'clock on a morning early in June. I heard the jingle of the bell on the bathroom door, which meant that he was up. I rushed to him as he stood, pondering, with his hand on the doorknob, fully dressed but in his stockinged feet, as he had slept, with his cap on his head. I helped him by lowering his beltless pants, underwear, and the diaper pad which was held in place by elastic straps.

"I have one here," he said, fiddling with his pants as he sat, trying to button them. "I have to finish it."

"You stay here," I told him, and waited nearby until I heard the tinkle of water and smelled the results of his bowel movement.

"I have to get up," he said. "I can't." He grasped the doorknob for support and tugged his heavy body to a bent but standing position.

"Hold on here," I said, indicating the opposite ledge, where he could lean while I cleaned him off. Patiently he waited, without trying to abort my efforts this time by pulling up his pants too soon.

Sometimes, when I took Grandpa to the toilet, he acted as though his privacy was being invaded; at other times, he was oblivious to what was happening. He stood, patiently, while I used rolls of toilet tissue to clean him off. If it took too long, he'd let me know, yanking at his pants and backing toward the wall. Once he tried to sit back down on the toilet, pinning me under him, but I forced him up and got out of the way.

Poor man! What recourse did he have? Mike said to me, "He knows he doesn't have much [control] left, but he's not giving up; not yet."

Everything in place, he shuffled to the table and chair where he sat, quiet and content, looking at anything and seeing nothing. I prepared his oatmeal with bran and milk and sugar and placed it before him. "Thank you, thank you," he said, reaching for my hand. Drawing it to his mouth, he kissed it thoroughly and profusely, his thanks and gratitude overflowing.

"You're welcome, Grandpa." I patted his back gently. Finally, he released my hand. His eye caught upon the doll gazing at him with her frozen smile from the table. It was the little-girl doll resurrected for him from the limbo of Cindy's closet.

"See? She's sitting, looking."

"I know," I replied, picking up the doll and moving it out of his reach. I left him to eat his oatmeal alone, because it was best that way, and I could monitor him from the next room.

When I returned, his oatmeal was half gone. He was holding the doll's arm in his left hand as he "fed" her. There was oatmeal on top of her orange hair, in her blue painted eyes, and dribbling down cheeks and chin onto her polka-dot dress.

"I give it to her," he explained.

"Yes, I see. Thank you!"

The doll was easily laundered and put away for a while, and Grandpa returned to playing with his dish. He wasn't very hungry this morning.

In June, Milt and I were privileged to baby-sit with each of our grandsons on different occasions. Shawn, now one year old, cried when he heard Grandpa's loud voice. He would follow him curiously from a distance with his eyes, but he didn't want to get close. When asked, "What does Great-Grandpa say?" he would answer, "My, my," with a serious expression, looking to see where Grandpa was.

Eric was too young to notice Grandpa at all. At three months of age, he slept most of the time, but Milt charmed him completely by bouncing him in his arms and making kissing sounds, causing him to smile and laugh. Being grandparents was wonderful. Both of us were happy to baby-sit whenever we could, but it didn't happen very often. Both of us had to be at home to do it; it was too hard for one of us to watch both Grandpa and a small child.

Another summer bonus was that there were frequent visits from Marian and Pat together, so that we could get to know both of the boys and they could become familiar with each other. Marian's six-month maternity leave would end with the last day of August, when Pat also would be returning to her job as a second-grade teacher.

Terese came home for one week in early June, after completing a training session at the "Y" camp in Michigan. She would be taking campers on group trips this year, planning for their food and activities together with an experienced leader. She was looking forward to this new experience. We hadn't seen Terese for months, since she had come home from school and left for camp while we were in France. She so seldom had time at home now; it was great visiting with her. One week though, was hardly enough for her to make contact with her many friends. I found myself repeating an archaic question: "When are you going to have time to straighten your room?" That was far down on her list of priorities. Life was far too exciting to waste on menial tasks.

Mike spent the summer as a camp counselor in Wisconsin. It was a change from his previous day camp jobs. He had a cabin full of seven-to-ten-year-olds under his charge, whom he had to entertain and keep from strangling one another as he tried to teach them a few things about nature. He learned a lot about the basic needs of children and what happens when they feel unloved and unwanted. His stories about some of their exploits and the tricks played on campers and counselors made it sound like a summer of fun.

Cindy was putting in as many hours as she could at the gas station, increasing her savings. She also spent considerable time at the piano and contending with an on-again, off-again relationship with a boyfriend. During July she took two weeks to attend a music camp for the study of the piano at the University of Illinois in Champaign. She had been asked to accompany the concert choir at the high school this year (her senior year), and she hoped this extra study would help her to prepare for it. One day my friend Jane came very early in the morning to stay with Grandpa while Milt, Cindy, and I drove to Champaign and saw Cindy registered and settled in a dormitory room with another young pianist. Milt and I then had lunch and returned to Chicago and O'Hare airport just in time to put Milt on a plane to Florida, where he attended a one-week principals' conference.

Later in July, Milt and I drove to Green Bay, Wisconsin, for a weekend visit with Mart, meeting his friends and witnessing his Pentecostal church in action. Mart played piano (by ear) for their rousing services and was very much committed to their way of life. Gone was the long hair, the sloppy look. Instead he was clean-shaven and neat, wearing suits and ties—albeit purchased at garage sales or thrift stores. He had decided to go back to school in the fall, to study mechanical engineering.

At the end of the month, Milt embarked by train on his now-annual backpacking trip, this time with four friends from the school district, to the Arapaho Mountains in Colorado. It was a magnificent trip full of great camaraderie.

This year the Christian Writers' Conference was scheduled for the week in mid-August when Milt had to be back at work. Fortunately for me, Jane was available to be with Grandpa every day during Milt's working hours, so I was able to go to Green Lake. My journey this year did not produce much in the way of poetry, but it was productive in another way. I was struggling with a decision: Do I really want to write a book about Grandpa? If so, how do I go about it?

A "Book Seminar" offered on the first day by a magazine editor provided helpful, step-by-step instructions. He challenged us to delve deep to ask ourselves why we wanted to write, then to do it, and to keep on—for ourselves, for the world, for God.

During the rest of the week, I wrestled with my conflicting feelings of fear and hope—fear that I would fail to write anything that would ever be published, fear of humiliation, of inadequacy, of lack of time, of my own pride; hope that I could achieve my goal. I explored those fears in depth and succeeded in putting them behind me, encouraged by my instructor and classmates. I returned home newly inspired to devote even more time to my writing project. Instead of spending three hours a week at the library, I asked Jane to come from nine until four every Thursday. It wasn't nearly enough, but it was a greater commitment. I now had to explain to people what I was doing, where I was. That made me more vulnerable. Milt invited me to have lunch with him each week. It was our "date" together and became a special time for us. He was interested in and supportive of my writing.

Throughout the summer Cindy had been more aloof than usual. Because her working hours were variable, she often worked through the dinner hour, eating her meals alone when it was convenient for her, and keeping to herself—either at the piano or in her room—at other times. It was her poems that called our attention to the fact that these were signs of dejection and un-happiness.

She would occasionally ask if I'd like to read a poem or two that she had just written, and I enjoyed having her confidence because I knew from my own experience how threatening it could be to share a poem—a piece of oneself—with another person. One poem described a young boy's suicide. This didn't surprise me too much, since I knew that Cindy was very sensitive to things going on around her. Later, however, she shared this poem and others on the themes of suicide and depression with her aunt Pat, who had come from Texas for a brief visit. My sister is a remarkably wise person, especially with young people. She alerted Milt and me immediately to the fact that Cindy might be in need of counseling. Milt had a list of counselors that he rec-ommended to parents of schoolchildren. When we had a chance to ask Cindy about going to see one of these counselors, she passed it off as unnecessary and unimportant, but she did agree to see one.

I made the arrangements with a woman Milt knew to be very competent. When I told Cindy about it, she became very angry and upset. "I'm not going! I'm not crazy!" she shouted, and ran stomping off up the stairs to her room. When she calmed down, I explained that no one thought she was crazy, but that it might be helpful for her to have someone to talk with. She finally agreed to go, on the condition that she would meet this person alone (no family sessions) and that no one else would know about it. Milt drove her to the office the first time; after that she went by herself.

I mention this only because I have some feelings that somehow Cindy might have been harmed by all of the friction, the arguments, the disharmony that peaked in our family after Grandpa's arrival. She was the youngest, and at ages eleven to sixteen, the most impressionable. Maybe her insecurity had nothing to do with Grandpa. I don't know. She was, however, the only one of the six who was present in our home during the entire time Grandpa stayed with us. Milt and I did our best to solve each problem and to weather this storm together as a family, but we knew that we were far from perfect. Just as we wanted to give Grandpa the kind of care he had every right to, whatever that might be, we wanted the same for our children. I am very thankful that I was made aware of Cindy's need for a kind of help she was not getting from us. It took a long time (two years in all) before Cindy had gained the self-confidence she needed for a healthy, vigorous outlook on life. Maybe she would have made it without outside help, but then again, maybe she would not. It feels good to be on the safe side of those maybe's.

Terese returned from summer camp with two whole weeks to prepare for her next adventure. She had applied to be, and had been accepted as, a volunteer on a work crew at a camp called "Farm and Wilderness" in Vermont. It is a place where city school-children stay for short periods to experience farm life and a more primitive lifestyle. Terese would spend two and a half months caring for farm animals, seeing them butchered or sold at auction, and working with young adults from many different back-grounds. She would sleep in a three-sided shelter and absorb some of the Quaker philosophy. She was in no hurry to get her college degree but was learning new things all the time, stretching herself and her horizons.

Cindy, for an early assignment in one of her fall classes, was required to make a "persuasive speech." She wanted to talk about her grandfather. How could she make it persuasive? she wanted to know. I gave her my file of information on Alzheimer's disease, and she finally decided on her title: "Keeping the Grandparent with Senile Dementia in the Home." She made graphs and charts for use on an overhead projector showing the percentage of people over age sixty-five who have senile dementia and the number of people in the United States who suffer from the disease. She emphasized that caring for such a person could be very frustrating and upsetting for the rest of the family, but that the benefits were worth the effort. She used pictures and gave examples from her own experience. She used the following passage from the book *The 36-Hour Day.*

One family member who attempted suicide said, "Looking back, I don't know why I felt that way. Things have been hard, but I'm glad I didn't die. My perceptions must have been all mixed up."*

She concluded with this statement: "I hope that what I've shared with you will make you more inclined, if you're ever in a similar situation, to welcome a victim of senile dementia into your home, realizing that although it will be difficult, all those involved can benefit."

Perhaps at this time Cindy was beginning to realize that her own perceptions had been "all mixed up" too. The speech was a success. She got an "A."

It was fall, and days were quieter for Grandpa and me. "I have to go home," he said determinedly one day. I was chopping vegetables to make stew for our evening meal. Stopping long enough to look at him, smile, and nod my head, I went on with my chopping, while he got up from his chair and began shuffling past me. He was heading for the "off limits" part of the house— the dining room and living room, where family newspapers, mail, and other possessions needed protection from Grandpa's "helpful" hands. I followed him and stood nearby, waiting to see whether he would take anything.

He went toward the picture window, reached behind the sheer

*Mace and Rabins, *The 36-Hour Day,* p. 179.

drape and down where he could see the sill, ran his hand along it. Perhaps he thought it was a door he could go through. Failing to find anything, he turned to the table, straightened the mail pile, and picked up a few envelopes from the top.

"Thank you, Grandpa," I said, reaching for them. Taking him by the hands as if he were a child, I tried to lead him back to the kitchen.

"You take everything!" he said, very offended, pulling away from me.

"Come on back, Grandpa," I urged verbally, prodding him physically at the same time.

"No, I won't."

Taking the tempting mail pile from the table, I left him alone but kept an eye on him as he shuffled around the table, moved a chair out of his way, and proceeded into the living room. Finding some pieces of wood in the bucket beside the fireplace, he studied them carefully before selecting a piece; then, seeing me waiting there, he offered one to me. I took it and placed it back in the bucket. He took a smaller piece, the size of a blackboard eraser. Satisfied with that, he went around to the dining room window again and began using the "eraser" to "clean" the window sill and wall beneath. Tiring of that, he wandered back to the kitchen. "I want to go home," he said again, and this time he headed for the door.

Later I added an introspective note in my journal:

Autumn Reverie

Autumn is getting to me. It has just about always been my favorite time of year. The sky is a vivid blue today, with scattered puffs of clouds that occasionally gang up and shut out the sun, sending a brisk, chilling breeze.

It's the autumn of my life. I've been thinking about that so much. So many sights of autumn—the leaves quaking in their brittleness, drifting, one by one; the intense blue, red-gold, and green of the landscape; the raw wind from the north; frost on the rooftops and sad, unripe tomatoes in the garden.

And here I am, after a happy spring, a lush, full summer. Why am I melancholy, nursing wounds of self-pity, dissatisfaction, inadequacy? Why am I sad, like the tomatoes?

One Sunday morning while Milt and I were at church, Cindy was sitting with Grandpa. As she sat, she wrote the following description while he ate his breakfast:

CINDY'S STORY: EATING OATMEAL

Grandpa is alone at the table—oblivious to my presence. He is very busy eating oatmeal. With his left hand he is turning the bowl, while his right hand, clutching a spoon, carefully pushes all of the oats from the edge of the bowl. He has noticed me and grunts his recognition. He raises the spoon, heaping with oats, to his mouth. The toothless gums frantically work up and down. His gray hair is a little curly because it has just been washed. He rubs his brow and smoothes his still damp hair as he chews. He makes soft noises—like humming noises, but short, like grunts. His face, in need of a shave, is creased with many wrinkles, but it is calm and placid. He looks at me, smiles, nods, and stares into space again until he has finished chewing. He is all alone in his thoughts. He again notices me and wordlessly offers me his last bite. He smiles and almost chuckles at my refusal. The spoon squeaks as it scrapes the empty bowl, but still the gums are working. The chewing motion does not stop. He frowns into the bowl, looking for the last morsel of oats. Everything is in slow motion except the jaws—they are out of place with the silent old man using all of his concentration to eat oatmeal. The bowl is now definitely empty, but he does not stop scraping it. It has become a habit. The spoon and the gums work together.

He is finished now. He rubs his hands and holds them as if they are cold. He wipes his nose on his sleeve. He nods his head with the jaw muscles finally at rest. He looks about in wonder. He looks outside. He sees something flying, he tells me. The jaws begin again as he tries to express himself with words that have left him long ago.

As the days grew shorter, Grandpa's bedtime habits worsened. He simply could not settle down and sleep. Three and four nights per week, he would be in and out of bed, talking loudly in nonsense syllables for an hour or even two hours at a time, being taken to the bathroom at intervals, beyond nine, ten and even eleven o'clock.

Getting him up early in the morning seemed a logical countermeasure, except that it didn't work. He sat in his chair and dozed, ignoring his food, his papers, everything, all morning.

In October we took him to see the neurologist again and asked for a change of medication. Doctor James suggested instead that we continue using the same tranquilizing drug but increase the dosage. He prescribed accordingly, outlining the minimum and maximum dosage to use. If that was ineffective, he said, he would prescribe a different drug.

We began with one pill per night, which was an increase over the previous dosage. For a few evenings there was no problem. Was the pill effective, or was Grandpa being good? The answer came when Grandpa's bedtime behavior reverted to what it had been before. We increased the dosage to two pills per night regularly, with a third pill when we became desperate, after ten or eleven o'clock at night. It was difficult to know whether the third pill finally knocked him out or whether he was exhausted by then and would have slept anyway.

In the morning, when I woke him, he sat in his chair and dozed, failing to become really awake until almost noon. Then he was insatiably hungry and restless, working up to his hyper behavior toward evening, and repeating the same cycle day after day.

This might have continued indefinitely, except that around Thanksgiving Day I noticed that Grandpa's right shoe was harder to get on his foot. When we showered him on the weekend, we noticed that his foot was swollen. Grandpa didn't complain at all. I soaked the foot in warm water a few times, hoping that the swelling would go down. It didn't, and the next weekend when we showered him again, we could see that the swelling was worse. By the middle of that week, Grandpa began to indicate there was pain in his foot. He refused to put any weight on his right foot and would only walk where there was something to hold on to. He was still groggy for half the day, then restless and hungry, then tired and sleepy; but he would talk at length when put to bed.

I thought that the pills, in the larger dosage we had been administering, might be a factor in these developments. I mentioned this to Milt, and we agreed to stop the medication entirely, for an indefinite period.

Meanwhile, Grandpa became steadily more inclined to sleep much of the day, sitting in his chair. Now he slept most of the night also, except when we took him to the bathroom in response to his talking.

Taking Grandpa to the bathroom became a major production now, because he could not help himself up, and his 145 pounds were a dead weight. It took two people to lift him. In a matter of three or four days, his vitality had visibly deteriorated. Even his ability to feed himself was lessened. He became sloppy, unable to handle a spoon effectively. I wondered if this was the crisis that would mark the end of home care for Grandpa.

Terese returned from Vermont, exuberant about her experiences there. She planned to go back in January. Meanwhile she got a job selling Christmas trees by persuading the store manager that she wanted to work outside in the cold, not at a cash register (in spite of being a female).

When Terese discovered that Grandpa had a sore foot, she was very upset with me for not taking him to the doctor. At this point I was not convinced that it was necessary.

We began using the wheelchair that we'd kept for such an emergency, so Grandpa went from bed to wheelchair to bathroom, back to chair, and to his bed at night. He dozed in the chair and had difficulty focusing his attention long enough to eat more than a few bites of food at a time. I consulted my sister Betty, the nurse. She said there was a possibility that Grandpa's swollen foot was due to a circulatory condition such as blood clots or congestive heart failure, but there was also a chance that he had fractured a bone in the ankle or foot. In order to clarify the situation I called Dr. James, who agreed to look at Grandpa right away.

Getting Grandpa from the wheelchair into our car was quite a task. At the hospital to which we had been directed to take him, an able attendant helped Milt lift Grandpa from the car to the hospital wheelchair. From there we took him to the doctor's consultation office and later to the X-ray department. Grandpa was passive, dozing much of the time, occasionally waking and saying, "My, my."

Our doctor observed Grandpa briefly, as did an internist who was with him. They both agreed that the swelling was probably due to lack of circulation rather than a broken bone. However, an X-ray was taken to be sure.

Dr. James suggested that we hospitalize Grandpa for a couple of days of testing and then place him in a nursing home because of the difficulty we were having with lifting him at home. The doctor assured us that he would not recommend any aggressive life-sustaining measures.

We returned home, and as we discussed the situation, Milt said that it was up to me to decide whether we should keep Grandpa at home or send him to a hospital or nursing home.

As I thought about this, I considered the possibility of Grandpa lingering for months in a semiconscious, bedridden state, requiring bed baths and feeding and extensive nursing care. I felt inadequate to provide this kind of care. I had never wanted to be a nurse and had no knowledge of the skills involved or interest in learning them. I felt that perhaps the time had come to put Grandpa into an institution where skilled people would do for him what I couldn't do.

I made a list of nursing homes and began calling them. It was very discouraging to learn the complex procedures involved. There were so many "levels of care," interviews required, forms to be filled out, and . . . waiting lists. (Of course, Dr. James had said he could place him, but that might be far away.)

After a few of these calls, I consulted with my sister again, describing Grandpa's condition to her, his grogginess, his lack of appetite and difficulty swallowing, which were evidence of continuous regression day by day.

Betty had cared for both of our parents in their last illnesses. Our mother and father had died peacefully at home under her care. She suggested that we keep Grandpa at home. She said he wouldn't linger long if he would not take food or drink.

With Betty's assurance that "you can handle it, Rosalie," I decided not to pursue the hospital and nursing home route, but at Betty's further suggestion Milt and I visited a medical equipment shop and rented a hospital bed and patient lift. The bed was a great help because it allowed us to raise Grandpa's head or legs for greater ease in feeding him and making him comfortable. (The lift was somewhat awkward, but we did use it to turn him in bed.) At this point, Grandpa remained in bed all the time.

During these days Grandpa was so quiet and was sleeping so much that we had to remind ourselves to go to him, to give him a few sips of juice or a few bites of food, or to talk to him. He would respond each time in a limited way, sometimes just opening his eyes, other times trying to say a few words. Frequently he would say, "Thank you," and would manage a smile. Then his eyes would glaze over and he would be sleeping again.

Christmas came in the middle of these changes. My sister did not join us for the holiday, nor did Pat and John, because Shawn was sick. Mart had a serious girlfriend and was invited to her home in Wisconsin. It was a quiet day with just Mike, Terese, Cindy, Marian, Jim, and little Eric, almost a year old, completing our holiday table. Grandpa remained in bed. He took only a few bites of food and a few sips of liquid from a spoon. Eric was cute in his red and white romper, able to stand and walk with help but not quite ready to take off on his own.

The day after Christmas, Mike went skiing and winter camping with a friend; Milt stayed home to help with Grandpa. The whole family would be together on New Year's Day, Grandpa's birthday, except for Terese, who planned to go to a YMCA winter camp session.

Grandpa's condition seemed to stabilize for a couple of days, but then the regression continued. Mike came home from his ski trip and went in to see Grandpa, as he always did when he had been away. He said he wondered if Grandpa still knew him, because he appeared to be completely gone. He fed him a few spoonfuls of applesauce, then held his hand awhile. "Do you recognize me?" he asked.

Incredibly, Grandpa looked at him, as if surprised, and said, "I reco'nize you."

On New Year's Eve, Grandpa would eat no solid food at all. He took a few spoonfuls of juice in the afternoon. As I stood there, urging him to open his mouth for more, I noticed that his eyes were open for several minutes. He was turned on his side and wasn't looking directly at me, but I felt that he could see me. His eyes seemed to be moist. He looked sad and thoughtful.

Later that evening Milt helped me turn him to his back, change his pad, and prop his knees up with pillows to make him more comfortable. We raised both the head and the foot of the bed so he was in a reclining position. He moaned when we turned him; otherwise he seemed to be in no pain.

CINDY'S STORY: GRANDPA DIED LAST NIGHT

It was New Year's Eve. I watched my mom spoon-feed Grandpa some apple juice. She was all dressed up, ready to go to a party at our church. I had been looking forward to being with my boyfriend that night, but when he came to my house, he said he was not feeling well and he would not be able to stay very long. He left around eight o'clock. My brother had already left to go to a party, too, so I was home alone (except for Grandpa, but he was in bed asleep). The time really dragged by. I watched television for a while, but I was very lonely. At around eleven thirty, I decided to play the piano to get some of my aggression out. As I was pounding out a song, I briefly considered whether or not I would wake Grandpa up. I doubted it because he was hard of hearing, but I really was not very concerned about him. At twelve o'clock midnight, I called my boyfriend, as planned, to wish him a happy new year. He was in bed, asleep, so his sleepy father told me. I went to bed very lonely and upset.

In the morning I was awakened by my mother, who was gently nudging me. "What do you want?" I snapped at her. "Grandpa died during the night," she said quietly. "I thought you would want to know. Your dad is calling the funeral home now." She left me to the quiet of my room. I lay in bed and cried. I kept thinking how I was the only one who could have been there to hold his hand when he died, but I was busy feeling sorry for myself. "Today is his birthday," I thought to myself. "He is (was) eight-nine years old." I wondered if we would still celebrate his birthday. As I lay there, I listened to my dad talking on the phone: talking to the funeral director, talking to my sister Marian and my sister Pat, trying to call my brother Martin (he wasn't home), and talking to my sister Terese, who was at winter camp. Terese wanted someone to take a picture of Grandpa. At that point I stopped listening to cry some more.

After a while, I got up, washed my tear-stained face, blew my nose, and ventured downstairs. Things had quieted down. My brother Mike was at church. My mom was on the phone talking to someone. I wanted to see Grandpa one more time, but I was scared. I went to the door of his room and opened it slowly. The bed was empty. They had already taken his body away. I was disappointed but also relieved. Later that afternoon, we did have the birthday dinner as planned. For us, of course, not for Grandpa. He would not have appreciated it anyhow.

The following day, Mike and I put together a chronological photo album of Grandpa. Terese and then Martin returned home.

At the wake, we put the photo album on display. There were lots of people there. Most of them had not known Grandpa personally but had heard stories about him. My nephew Shawn, not yet two years old, was there running around. He had already learned that

"Great-Grandpa is with God in heaven." Towards the end
of the evening, I got up enough nerve to go to the coffin.
What I saw both surprised and bothered me. I had
thought he would look like he was sleeping, but it did
not look like him at all. When he was alive, his hands
were all red and blue from clotted blood, but now they
were chalk white. His mouth was closed, too, but he
never slept with his mouth closed. I had never seen him
lying flat on his back either. As I was studying this
strangely unfamiliar body, my dad came over to me and
gave me a hug.

The next day, at the funeral, I held Shawn on my lap
while Pat, his mother, walked up the aisle as a pallbearer.
Later in the service I sang harmony to one of the songs
with the woman who did the music for the service. Mike
gave the eulogy after that and spoke about some things
he had learned from having Grandpa with us. Afterward,
at the grave site, my brother Mart spoke about his memories of Grandpa. I stood and watched as the coffin was
lowered into the frozen ground, feeling my toes grow
numb to the cold. After a while, I could not even feel the
snow wedged between my nearly bare toes. We threw
roses on the coffin before we left.

As I walked away I realized that the part of Grandpa
that made him special, the Grandpa that I loved, had
been dead weeks before his heart actually stopped beat-
ing. I realized, also, that he would never really be dead
because he is alive in my memories, which I carry with
me wherever I go.

The day after Grandpa's death, I wrote some thoughts about
his time with us in my journal:

Different Ways of Loving
    People love in different ways. That's evident to me
right now as I see the different ways we in the family
loved Grandpa.
    I always thought I didn't love him. Now I realize that I

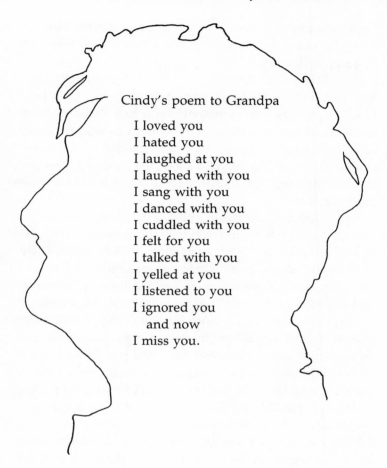

Cindy's poem to Grandpa

I loved you
I hated you
I laughed at you
I laughed with you
I sang with you
I danced with you
I cuddled with you
I felt for you
I talked with you
I yelled at you
I listened to you
I ignored you
 and now
I miss you.

did. I loved him primarily by caring for his physical needs, by giving him my time and my energy, but also by trying to understand and accept him, never quite making it, never quite coming to the point where I wanted to tell him that I loved him, or actually feeling love for him in my own heart.

Milt loved him as a son, verbalizing his love often by telling Grandpa that he loved him and saying "God bless you" when he tucked him into bed at night. He loved him by spending time with him, holding his hand, sitting quietly; and by putting up with the frustrations, ministering to his physical needs, providing a home for him when he needed it, forgiving him for failing to love him more or better as a father.

Mike loved Grandpa for himself, for his capacity to live, to laugh, to respond, to be whatever he could be. Mike's love was unconditional, yet it had its limits insofar as he could not minister to Grandpa's physical needs to any great extent. His was more of a response to a psychological need, but he gave Grandpa as much attention as he could and was a strong advocate in his favor whenever possible.

Terese loved Grandpa in still another way. She responded to the child in Grandpa, the frivolous, unsophisticated joy and simplicity she found in him, particularly in the early stages of his illness. It was difficult for her to pay attention to him when he lost full human awareness and withdrew into a shell of pure physical existence.

Cindy loved him in a more objective way, I think. She related to him as a fellow human being needing love, attention, and affirmation. She resented his difficult ways in the early years of his being in our home, when his demands conflicted with her own needs for attention, time, and space; but she recognized his need to be loved and responded to that need whenever she could.

Mart was here so seldom that he was touched very little by Grandpa's presence, yet he was challenged in the early years by Grandpa's insults and demands. Mart's response was typically quiet withdrawal. He never showed any anger or resentment, and his love was one of acceptance of Grandpa's right to be here. He supported us in our care of Grandpa and all that it entailed, and on a few occasions he stayed with Grandpa when we went somewhere; but Mart kept his distance and didn't want to be too involved.

Marian and Pat loved Grandpa from a distance too, since they visited our home only occasionally, and since they had really lost touch with him during the nine years of his widowhood when he lived alone. Their love was expressed in their support for our decision to care for Grandpa at home rather than to put him into a nursing home. They ministered to him whenever an occasion came up and we asked for their help. This was in reverence for his position as a grandparent, and out of respect for him as an aged person.

I suppose love has as many different expressions as there are persons. A line from a song comes to mind, one that was popular when I was young and became part of my basic philosophy of life:

The greatest thing
You'll ever learn
Is just to love
And be loved
In return.*

---

*"Nature Boy," popularized by a Nat King Cole recording. Words and music by Eden Ahbez. Copyright 1946, 1948 by Crestview Music Corp., Capitol Records, New York, New York.

Postscript

Some weeks later we received a neuropathology report from the surgeon who performed an autopsy of Grandpa's brain after his death. It confirmed the fact that Grandpa did have Alzheimer's disease.

Gradually the house regained its normalcy: the rented hospital bed and lift were returned, pictures were put back on the walls, the bell was removed from above the bathroom door. Grandpa's clothing was sorted and placed in boxes to be given away; his little "saw table" which he had built years ago as a cabinet, now with the scrapes and gouges made by clamp and saw during those years of his wood cutting—this was first put outside to be discarded, later reclaimed as a relic. Terese, Mike, and Cindy kept some of the items that were meaningful to them: his caps, his pipes.

The traces of Grandpa's presence were disappearing, yet we encountered him everywhere. When Milt made a loud noise in clearing his throat I gave a start, thinking for a split second that it was Grandpa's voice. We found ourselves saying, "My, my!" with knowing smiles at one another. When Cindy and I planned to shop for some clothing on a Sunday afternoon, Milt made a mental note that he would stay home while we were gone. It wasn't until later that he realized that he didn't have to stay home; he was free to go to the office to do some extra work. When Milt and I drove together on a Saturday to do some special shopping, we both confessed to having the feeling that "we must hurry home to take care of Grandpa." That feeling persisted for a long time.

The gradual languishing of Grandpa's body during that last half-year or so, coupled with my increasing church involvements and my days at the library writing about this experience, had caused me to be away from home so much that I told Jane it seemed she was spending more time with Grandpa than I was. Therefore my life didn't stop suddenly with Grandpa's death. I had already gone on to new things. Writing about Grandpa's years with us caused me to relive them constantly, but that was therapeutic, and I enjoyed the challenge.

Mike found a teaching position and moved to Chicago in August to begin his new independent life. Cindy enrolled as a freshman honors student at Northern Illinois University, later to choose a major in family counseling. Terese decided to pursue a career as a dentist and returned to school in earnest. She transferred to the University of Illinois at Champaign. Milt and I began to relish being "just the two of us" for the first time in thirty-two years. We enjoyed a marvelous trip to England and Ireland that summer.

We felt at once sad and happy to know that Grandpa was gone—at peace at last. We missed him; he was a large part of our lives. But we had few regrets. We had done what we could for him, often more than we wanted to do. It was a decision we carried out together, Milt and I, as many labors of love are done: sometimes joyfully, sometimes guiltily, sometimes dutifully or resentfully, but gladly, all the same. Now we remembered the love that permeated the entire experience, that motivated it, that challenged us continually, and that brought us through the trial successfully.

Becoming a caretaker of a person with Alzheimer's disease is a devastating experience. I believe, however, that it is within the power of the human spirit to draw from that experience something good, something of beauty, like the geranium, plucked at the peak of its summer radiance, and Grandpa's words:

Here's something
something good.
You take it.

JOURNEY WITH GRANDPA

Designed by Martha Farlow.

Composed by Capitol Communications, in Palatino.

Printed by R. R. Donnelley & Sons Company on 50-lb. Cream White Sebago and bound in Joanna Arrestox A.